PREFACE AND INTROD

The Multi-Specialty Recruitment Assessment (MSRA) is
process of General Practice (GP) and other run-through specialties. Some candidates sitting
the paper have a strong background in their general medicine, but more often than not, may
lack the knowledge required for certain subspecialties including obstetrics and gynaecology
and paediatrics.

This book provides a concise review of essential topics that may be tested in the MSRA
exam. This would allow prospective candidates to have a rapid review of topics, taking
revision pressure off in the face of busy clinical schedule. Importantly, candidates sometime
fail to realise that the MSRA is designed as a GP knowledge examination and may over-
revise. This is not helped by online question banks, which do not tailor their questions. These
questions often feel like a copy-and-paste from other examination format, resulting in a vast
amount of irrelevancy. This book aims to address this by focusing on relevant as well as
challenging topics, allowing one to separate the tress from the forest of knowledge.

There are no pictures in the actual exam, and actual descriptions of a condition are used
instead. This book is written to reflect that. NICE/National guidelines are also summarised.

This book may be suitable for medical students as a revision aid for their Internal Medicine
rotation or Finals.

We hope you find this book useful.

B.N.
J.H.

HOW TO USE THIS BOOK

- This is the first book out of two in the series. It only covers medical concepts.
- This book does not cover the Situation Judgement Test part of the MSRA.
- This book is not a comprehensive text for the entirety of medicine – it only highlights
  high-yield points and information that are commonly missed (even in Question
  Banks).
- It should be supplemented by a main text and practice questions.

CHAPTER LIST

1. CARDIOLOGY

GENERAL TIPS
- Ensure that you know the descriptive terms for ECG findings (no diagrams in the exam)

- Resuscitation UK algorithm should be memorised

- Indications, side effects and interactions of cardiology medications always appear in the exam.

INTERVENTIONAL CARDIOLOGY

Stable angina
- Exertional cardiac-sounding chest pain; relieved by PRN GTN
- CT coronary angiogram (CTCA) is the NICE-approved 1st line investigation
  - **Stress testing (exercise tolerance) is NEVER THE ANSWER for angina testing.**
- NICE algorithm
  - Step 1: beta blocker (BB). Caution in asthmatics. E.g. atenolol/bisoprolol
  - Step 2: and/or dihydropyridine calcium channel blockers (CCB) e.g. amlodipine or diltiazem
  (but 1st line for Prinzmetal angina)
  - Step 3: Add one of the following (usually 2 drugs max):

Isosorbide mononitrate modified release	Vasodilator. Should be given 0800 and 1400 – to allow nitrate-free period, avoiding nitrate intolerance. S/E: flushing, headaches, hypotension
Ivabradine Cardiac pacemaker inh.	Slows HR down. Patient needs to be in **normal sinus with resting HR ≥ 70 bpm**. Should be stopped in **3 months** if not working.
Ranolazine Inhibits Na⁺ in.	Helps with HR – so good choice if bradycardic S/E: long QT, avoid in moderate cardiac, renal, liver failures
Nicorandil Opens K⁺ channels	Vasodilator. C/I: low BP, LV dysfunction

  - Step 4: revascularisation
- Secondary prevention: aspirin 75 mg, statins; ACE-inhibitor if diabetic or LV dysfunction.

★ Prinzmetal angina = vasospasm, almost always at rest
(usually midnight - early morning).
can occur in clusters of 2-3.

CARDIOVASCULAR RISK AND LIPID MODIFICATION

Qrisk2 score – used to quantify 10-year cardiovascular risk (PRIMARY prevention)
Should be used every 5 years (unless already have cardiovascular disease or high risk or > 85y).
Statins are given **if** QRisk2 > 10% or if lifestyle interventions ineffective.
In > 85 y or patients with CKD, atorvastatin 20 mg may be used without risk stratification.

In proven CVD – high-intensity statins should be used for 2° prevention (e.g. 80 mg atorvastatin).
Target: **3 months > 40% non-HDL reduction.** If not achieved, aim higher dose.
S/Es: myositis (and rhabdomyolysis – rare), hepatitis, constipation
Monitoring: LFTs baseline, 3 months, 12 months.
DO NOT measure CK if asymptomatic.
Statins are contraindicated in pregnancy.
Amlodipine (weak inhibitor) interacts with simvastatin (increase level). Not the case for other
statins.

Ezetimibe – monotherapy of primary hypercholesterolaemia where statins are contraindicated.
Fibrates – used in secondary care. Better to reduce triglycerides. More risk of gallstones.
Combination of statins and fibrates increase risk of rhabdomyolysis.
Aliro/evoloCUmab – specialist drug for primary *heterozygous* familial hypercholesterolaemia to lower
LDL-C. Alirocumab - ↑ uptake of LDL - chlesterol.

Unstable angina and acute coronary syndromes
- Remember that **diabetics** may not experience chest pain.
- UA – cardiac-sounding chest pain at rest, **troponin negative**. GRACE score
  determines risk: if moderate or high (6m mortality > 3%) – angiogram +/- proceed in
  same admission within 72 hours. Low-risk → dual antiplatelet therapy (DAPT) +
  elective angiogram
- Prinzmetal angina and cocaine abuse
  - Cocaine toxicity – that of sympathetic stimulation
  - Coronary vasospasms – therefore no lesion to stent
  - Tx: nitrates (GTN) + CCB (diltiazem) +/- angiogram if not controlled; benzos
    to treat cocaine-induced hypertension
- ACS protocol: MONA-BASH   O₂ if sats < 94%.
  - Morphine, O2, nitrates (GTN SL)   morphine if severe pain.
  - Antiplatelets (DAPT)   Nitrates if ongoing pain | ↑BP.
    - Aspirin **chewed** PLUS   Ticagrelor unless ↑ bleeding risk.
    - Ticagrelor or clopidogrel
  - Secondary prevention: bisoprolol, ACE-inhibitor, statins
  - Heparin (in the form of fondaparinux) 12hrs
  - PPCI: door-to-balloon if STEMI: 90 minutes, NSTEMI: up to 72 hours
- ACS ECGs and differentials of ST/TW changes:
  - ST elevation > 1mm in 2 contiguous limb lead and > 2mm in 2 contiguous
    chest leads (1.5 mm in women)

GRACE score - age, HR, BP, cardiac (Killip class) e renal function (creat),
cardiac arrest on presentation, ECG findings, troponin.

Inferior	II, III, aVF changes → RCA/LCx
Anterior	V1, 2, 3, 4 changes → LAD
Lateral	I, aVL, V5, V6 changes → LCx/LAD Diagonal branch
Other red flags:	New BBB Biphasic T wave in V1 and V2 (Wellen's syndrome – critical LAD stenosis)
Pericarditis	Widespread concave ST elevation with PR depression Tx: NSAID, colchicine (S/E: D/N/V – as microtubule assembly inhibitor: targets active cells e.g. gut)
Brugada syndrome	Coved ST segment elevation in more than one of V1,2,3 Followed by T wave inversion → risk fatal arrhythmia.
Hypertrophic obstructive cardiomyopathy	Left ventricular hypertrophy – non-specific ST segment and T wave changes • Voltage criteria: modulus sum of deep S wave (negative deflection) in V1 + tall R wave (positive deflection) in V5-6 > 35 mm ↳ if strain • Non-voltage: ST depression, TWI in left-sided leads Asymmetrical deep septal hypertrophy – deep, narrow Q waves in lateral and inferior leads. Left atrial enlargement – P mitrale: double notched P waves
High take-off	Young, healthy men – widespread ST elevation at J point (junction between end of QRS and start of ST segment)

- ACS drugs:
  - Omeprazole interacts with clopidogrel (reduces its effectiveness as omeprazole is a P450 inhibitor and clopidogrel is a prodrug that requires liver activation) but **not** lansoprazole. Also, ticagrelor is not a prodrug and may be used instead.
  - Tirofiban – used in high-risk patient. Causes anaemia and thrombocytopenia
- DVLA advice:
  - ACS Group 1 – no need to notify; resume **1 week if successful Tx and LVEF ≥ 40% before discharge and no further revascularisation planned**
    - Otherwise: 4 weeks
  - ACS Group 2 (HGV) – notify; re-licensed **at least 6 weeks later** if LVEF ≥ 40%, ETT free of signs or ECG changes using Bruce protocol
  - Elective PCI Group 1 – 1 week; Group 2 – 6 weeks (+ notify).
- Complications of MI: timeline

< 4 hours	Cardiogenic shock and arrest, arrhythmias
4 – 24 hours	Arrhythmias
1 – 3 days	Fibrinous pericarditis
4 – 7 days	Rupture of free wall, interventricular shunt, papillar muscle rupture (= regurgitation)
Weeks to months	Fibrosis of ventricular wall = weak → aneurysms with mural thrombus; Dressler syndrome (autoimmune pericarditis); depression

HYPERTENSION

- Ambulatory BP monitoring (ABPM) is offered if BP between 140/90 -180/120 mmHg. It takes 2 measurements per hour between patient's waking hours.
- Alternatively, home BP monitoring (HBPM) can be used – seated patient, 2 measurements 1 minute apart, BD (morning and evening), and for 4-7 days.
- Dx criteria: clinical BP > 140/90 mmHg **and** A/HBPM average of > 135/80 mmHg.
  - Stage 1: 140-159/90-99 mmHg clinically **and** A/HBPM 135-149/85-94 mmHg
  - Stage 2: 160-179/100-119 clinically **and** A/HBPM 150/95 or higher
  - Stage 3: SBP > 180 or DBP >120 mmHg chronically (any method)
- NICE algorithm
  - Step 1:
    - < 55y or **T2DM** → ACE-inhibitor (ramipril)/ARB
    - ≥ 55y or Afro/Caribbean → CCB (amlodipine)
      - S/E: ankle oedema (local vasodilation), headache, flushing, *gingival hyperplasia*, constipation. Nifedipine causes ulcers.
  - Step 2:
    - < 55y or T2DM → ACE-inhibitor (ramipril)/ARB + CCB or ACE-inhibitor + thiazide-like diuretic (indapamide)
      - S/E thiazides: **impotence**, hypoNa/K, *hyper*Ca, precipitate gout (hyperuricaemia).
    - ≥ 55y or Afro/Caribbean → CCB (amlodipine) + ACE-inhibitor or CCB + thiazide-like diuretic
  - Step 3:
    - Common pathway → ACE-inhibitor + CCB + thiazide-like diuretic
  - Step 4:
    - Add on **spironolactone** if K+ ≤ 4.5
    - Add on BB or α–blocker if K+ > 4.5
- Red flags: < 40 years, sudden worsening, accelerated/malignant, stroke < 50 years, refractory (>140/90 mmHg or > 130/80 with DM/renal disease and on 3 different regimen including diuretic) – should investigate for **secondary causes of hypertension:**
  - Endocrine diseases
    - Acromegaly → OGTT and IGF-1 levels
    - Hyperthyroidism → TFTs
    - Conn's adenoma → aldosterone: renin ratio > 40 → CT adrenal → lateralisation (e.g. adrenal venous sampling)
      - Note ACE-I/ARB will decrease the ratio
    - Cushing's → low-dose dexamethasone suppression test
    - Phaeochromocytoma → 24h urinary metanephrines
  - Renal diseases
    - Adult polycystic kidney disease → US renal tract
    - Renal artery stenosis and fibromuscular dysplasia → MRA renal arteries +/- angiogram
    - Glomerulonephritis → dipstick, MCS, protein:
- Controlling blood pressure in special scenarios:
  - In systemic sclerosis renal crisis – **ramipril** is the drug of choice (directly interferes with pathophysiology pathway of scleroderma: hyperreninaemia from renal artery sclerosis)
  - Preeclampsia – IV magnesium sulphate

- o Aortic dissection – IV labetalol/esmolol (target nSBP 100-120 mmHg)
- o Conn's syndrome – spironolactone
- o Malignant hypertension – nitrates, nitroprusside, labetalol
- o Subarachnoid haemorrhage – nimodipine reduces vasospasm; hyperhydration (3L)

HEART FAILURE

- New York Heart Association classification: class I – not limitations; class IV – Sx at rest.
- Most common presentation are the "congested" patients (warm and wet) with known HF.
  - o Daily weights, fluid restrict, strict input and output chart, U&Es, and echo.
  - o Offloading IV diuretics e.g. **furosemide** 0800 and 1400 (to avoid diuresis at night), optimise other medications. Switching to PO **bumetanide**.
  - o If renal function is poor – can consider a combination of ISMN and hydralazine.

- Key drugs in heart failure with reduced ejection fraction (LVEF < 40%):

Furosemide	Loop diuretic to offload fluids. **No prognostic benefit.** S/E: hypoK/Na, exacerbation of hyperglycaemia and gout. Add K+-sparing diuretic (e.g. MRA); if refractory oedema consider thiazides (e.g. metolazone)
ACE inhibitors/ Angiotensin receptor blockers	**Prognostic benefit – helps remodel the heart by reducing afterload** S/E: hyperkalaemia, dry cough, angioedema ARB e.g. losartan can be considered if dry cough untolerated
Bisoprolol	**Prognostic benefit.** Caution in asthmatics; should not be used with non-dihydropyridine CCBs such as verapamil (causes low cardiac output). *Other beta blockers with prognostic benefits: Carvedilol (cardio-selective), metoprolol.* Beta-blocker overdose – treated with **glucagon**.
Mineralocorticoid antagonist (MRA) e.g. spironolactone	K+ sparing. **Prognostic benefit.** S/E: painful gynaecomastia (as spironolactone is non-selective and can block androgen receptors); hyperkalaemia; Selective aldosterone receptor antagonist e.g. eplerenone can be considered if sexual S/E intolerant: gynaecomastia or impotence
Entresto	Combination of valsartan (**prognostic benefit**) and sacubitril **Indications:** LVEF < 35%
Ivabradine	**Indications:** LVEF < 35% and normal sinus and HR > 75bpm
Digoxin	Loading due to long half-life. **Indications:** normal sinus rhythm to improve symptoms (+ve inotropy) such as AF and rest shortness of breath.

- Devices in heart failure:
  - Implantable cardiac defibrillator (ICD) – mainly used in cases of narrow complex QRS without LBBB
  - Cardiac Resynchronisation Therapy (CRT, biventricular pacing) – synchronously contract the ventricles to increase output. Used in patients with LBBB or broad QRS complexes ($\geq$ 150 ms), which indicate ventricular dysynchrony.
    - In NYHA IV – CRT-P (pacemaker) is used if LBBB/QRS width criteria met, as the patient is essentially in end-stage heart failure. If QRS < 120 ms – the only option is to optimise medical therapy.
    - In other NYHA classes, CRT-D (defibrillator) is generally used when criteria is met (option for CRT-P if NYHA class III).
- No prognostic medications for HF with preserved ejection fraction (HFpEF) – only management is diuretics for symptoms. In fact, medications like beta blockers slow down the heart – diminishing the only compensation (tachycardia) in HFpEF.
- Pulmonary oedema
  - A – sit patient up, CPAP; B – high-flow O_2
  - C – if SBP > **90-100** mmHg, can give nitrate (spray or infusion), nitroprusside, and opiates. Caution with furosemide (offload) and IV fluids (slow infusion).
  - D/E – treat underlying causes
  - Avoid beta blockers (negative chrono/inotropy).
  - If SBP < 90 mmHg persistently – treat as cardiogenic shock (require inotropes)
- High output heart failure – occurs in face of increasing needs e.g. anaemia, hyperthyroidism, Paget's, acromegaly, AV malformations, pregnancy, malnutrition.

VALVULAR ISSUES

Aortic stenosis
- Presents as angina, syncope, or SOB on exertion (5, 3, 1.5 years from symptoms to death respectively). Left heart failure and aforementioned Sx due to LV working too hard to pump blood across a narrow opening (LV outflow tract obstruction)
- Therefore, **bad drugs in severe AS:** (1) decrease afterload (vasodilators and ACE inhibitors – heart cannot pump out more blood to compensate for fall in systemic vascular resistance) , (2) decrease contractility (beta blockers, CCBs). Both can cause blood pressure to drop.
- Ejection systolic murmur loudest at left sternal edge, radiating to the carotids **(not present in aortic *sclerosis*)**; parvus et tardus (low-volume, slow-rising) pulse.
- Surgery if (1) symptomatic, or (2) asymptomic with severe stenosis
- Otherwise, monitoring with yearly echo
- **Do not do a stress exercise test.**

Mitral regurgitation
- Usually mild or asymptomatic but severe MR presents as heart failure (such as flash pulmonary oedema).
- As the regurgitant dilates the left atrium, there is predisposition to AF.
- Medical Tx is to thus control heart failure and AF.
- The circulation is hyperdynamic (apex displaced down with left parasternal heave)
- Apical pansystolic murmur radiating to the axilla.
- Stable and mild cases are monitored annually; severe cases require surgery.

Infective endocarditis
- *S. aureus* now most common bug.
- Transthoracic echo is most commonly used – but **gold-standard** is a transoesophageal one
- IVDU have right-sided **acute** endocarditis (tricuspid) due to venous introduction.
- Aortic valve vegetation → check ECG (PR interval prolongation) – monitor for abscess causing aortic root dilatation.
- Septic emboli to rich vascular beds e.g. kidneys → urine dipstick; brain → MRI; retina (Roth spots) → fundoscopy; splenomegaly → CTAP; acute limb ischaemia → pulses/
- *S. bovis* and other gut commensal isolated → **colonoscopy** to screen for colorectal cancer.
- **Duke criteria** – for definitive Dx: 2 major or 1 major + 3 minor or all minor criteria
  - **Major ("BE")** → Blood culture positive x2 (or culture/histology positive from vegetations removed); Endocardium involvement (new murmur, abscess etc.)
  - **Minor ("FEEVER")** → Fever > 38°C, Evidence cultures that don't meet major criteria, Evidence of immunological phenomenon (glomerulonephritis, Osler nodes), Vascular phenomenon (Janeway lesions, embolic), Risk factors (predisposing conditions, IVDU)
- **No antibiotics prophylaxis** for invasive procedures (including tattoos and piercing).
- **Differentials:**
  - Libmann-Sacks endocarditis – sterile vegetations on both side of valve in SLE

  - o Atrial myxoma – female with positional dizziness, SOB, palpitations with pansystolic murmur. Carney syndrome = systemic myxomas with endocrine disorder.

Carcinoid syndrome
- A combination of adult-onset refractory wheeze (mistaken for asthma), diarrhoea, facial flushing, and new murmur should alert you to this rare condition.
- In carcinoid syndrome, 5-HT (serotonin) is excessively being produced – causing these symptoms and valvular fibrosis (right-sided: pulmonary stenosis or tricuspid regurg).
- If the carcinoid tumour is in the bowel – there must be liver mets that will allow 5-HT to escape liver metabolism for the syndrome to occur. Carcinoid lung tumours do not need mets.
- Tx: octreotide (synthetic somatostatin) and resection

OTHER COMMONLY TESTED ECGs

There are no pictures in the MSRA – you need to get used to descriptors.

Bradycardia

First degree heart block	PR interval is prolonged only (> 200 ms), QRS relationship maintained
Mobitz I (Wenckebach)	PR interval is prolonged progressively until QRS is skipped "Grouped beating"
Mobitz II	PR interval normal Randomly skipped QRS complexes (can be wide)
Third degree (complete) heart block	AV dissociation – no relationship between P waves and QRS complexes
Bifascicular block	Right bundle branch block and Left anterior or posterior fascicular block **i.e. left** or **right** axes deviation respectively (in absence of other causes of deviation)
"Classical" trifascicular block	Bifascicular block and first degree heart block Misnomer – a true trifascicular block is a complete heart block…

Tachycardia

Monomorphic VT	Identical, repetitive morphology of broad QRS. Concordant (all up or down).
Polymorphic VT	Multiple morphology of broad QRS complexes of different amplitude axes, and duration. Concordant (all up or down).
Torsades de pointes	Polymorphic VT with long QT, with an axis that twist around an isoelectric baseline (therefore, discordant – alternating up then down) **Tx: Magnesium**
Ventricular fibrillation	Chaotic irregular waveforms of varying amplitude. No P/QRS/T.

Others

Tachy-brady syndrome	Alternating brady and tachycardia. **Tx:** pacemaker for bradycardia and rate-control (beta blockers) for tachy
Pulseless electrical activity	Any ECG rhythm (including sinus) BUT clinically no pulse
Wolf-Parkinson-White	Slurred upstroke of QRS complex (delta wave) PR interval is shortened
Arrhythmogenic right ventricular cardiomyopathy	Small positive deflection at the end of QRS (epsilon wave); slightly wide QRS.
Pericarditis	Widespread concave ST elevation and PR depression (except aVR – PR elevation). Later on, ST changes normalise with T waves inversions.
Hypothermia	Bradycardia w ventricular ectopic Prolongation of everything: PR, QRS, QT Positive deflection at the J point i.e. end of QRS, start of ST stegment – (Osborn (J) waves)
Hypercalcaemia	Short QT mainly

Hypocalcaemia	Long QT – can degenerate to torsades de pointes
Hyperkalaemia	Prolonged PR interval, small/absent P waves Peaked T waves Widened QRS complexes Eventually degenerate to sinusoidal rhythm → VF → asystole
Hypokalaemia	Deflection after the T wave (U wave) Flat T waves ST depression
Right bundle branch block	In V1-3– narrow RS complex with another large positive deflection called R' (RSR' wave), hence looks like an "M" (V1 is **UPright**)
Left bundle branch block	In V1-3 – deep downward deflecting S wave (QS or rS wave). Hence looks like "W".
Pacemaker rhythms	RV pacemaker will lead to LBBB (due to source of electricity starting from the right side and travelling across non-conducting tissues to left – left sided "blocked"). Vice-versa.
Pulmonary embolism	Most common ECG: **sinus tachycardia** Evidence of right heart strain: right axis deviation, ST depression and T wave inversion in V1-3, II, III, aVF (anteroinferior) Q wave in I, S and T wave inversion in III (Q1S3T3) is rare.

Causes of long QT: (1) drugs: DIGOXIN, TCA, macrolides, quinolones, anti-psychotics; (2) the 6 "hypos": hypokalaemia, hypomagnesaemia, hypocalcaemia, hypothermia, hypothyroidism, hypoadrenalism (Addison's); (3) ischaemia and general medical illness

trial fibrillation and flutter

- AF ECG: irregularly irregular QRS *narrow* complexes with lack of P waves
- Flutter ECG: P waves with sawtooth baseline, 300 bpm limited by AV blocks (for example – 2:1 block has 2 P waves per 1 QRS complex)
- Management: rate <u>or</u> rhythm control and anticoagulation; treat underlying cause
- To determine need of anticoagulation: calculate HASBLED and CHAD2S2VASc score – the female sex category only applies if there are any other score**
- Rate or rhythm controls depend on the patient – younger and reversible/acute onset < **48h** or Sx of CCF: try the latter.
- Rhythm control
    - o Electrical: DC cardioversion
        - Needs an echo to check intramural thrombus
        - Needs to be anticoagulated to prevent thrombus. For **4 weeks** and to continue *after* procedure for **12 months** or until advised by cardiology (due to myocardial stunning)
    - o Electrical: ablation (pulmonary vein)
    - o Chemical cardioversion
        - AmIODarone – preferred for patient with **LV failure**.
            - Needs loading dose as very long half-life
            - Dirty drug – many side effects: photosensitivity, slate-grey pigmentation, hepatotoxicity, thyroid (hypo/hyper – contains IODine), and pulmonary fibrosis
            - Interactions with **warfarin** and **digoxin**
        - Flecanide – for paroxysms (as a "pill in pocket"); **cannot be used in patients with structural heart condition**.
- Rate control
    - o Beta blockers (bisoprolol; acutely = metoprolol IV) – preferred if co-existing angina or hypertension
    - o Calcium channel blockers (diltiazem or verapamil)
    - o Digoxin – used in sedentary patients; only reduces ventricular rate *at rest*. Some positive inotropy – useful in CHF.
        - **Overdose**: N/V/D + blurred vision w xanthopsia/haloes + palpitations/syncope + confusion. Tx = Fab fragment to digoxin (Digibind)
    - o **Above drugs are not given if a patient has an accessory pathway (WPW – pre-excited AF) as it will favour conduction down that pathway (losing AV node safety netting)**

C – congestive HF
H – hypertension
A2 – age $\geq$ 75   +2
D – diabetes mellitus
S2 – stroke/TIA/VTE
V – vascular (MI, PVD)
A – age 65-74y
Sc – female sex **

EMERGENCIES

- **Adverse features:** shock, syncope, MI, HF
- **Profound bradycardia**
  - Atropine 500 mcg
  - → repeat up to 3 mg max *if* risk of asystole
    - Recent asystole, Mobitz II heart block or higher degree, pause > 3s.
  - → alternatives: transcutaneous pacing, IV isoprenaline, IV adrenaline
  - They would need a permanent pacemaker once stabilised
- **Unstable tachycardia**
  - Synchronised DC shock x3
  - Then amiodarone 300 mg IV 10-20 minutes
  - Then repeat shock
  - Then amiodarone 900 mg over 24h
- **Regular narrow complex tachycardia**
  - Use vagal manoeuvres
  - Adenosine 6/12/12 mg IV boluses
  - Rate control with beta blockers e.g. in flutter
- **Irregular narrow complex tachycardia**
  - Treat as fast AF – BB/CCB/digoxin/amiodarone
- **Regular broad complex tachycardia**
  - Amiodarone 300 mg IV (20-60 mins) then 900 mg over 24h loading
  - If SVT with aberrancy – give adenosine as per regular NCT protocol
- **Irregular broad complex tachycardia**
  - AF with BBB – treat as per NCT protocol
  - Pre-excited AF – amiodarone
  - Polymorphic VT/torsades – magnesium 2g over 10 minutes
- **Tamponade/large effusion**
  - Beck's triad: muffled heart sounds, raised JVP, hypotension
  - Other signs: Kussmaul's sign – paradoxically raised JVP on inspiration; pulsus paradoxus – exaggerated BP variation with respiratory cycle (inspiration leads to fall, vice-versa)
  - **ECG shows**: low voltage QRS complexes alternating in amplitude (height) – "electrical alternans" due to heart bringing back and forth in fluid-filled pericardium
  - Tx: IV fluids; pericardiocentesis

- **Anaphylaxis**
  - o Key drugs

Drug	Age	Dose
Adrenaline IM (1:1000, repeat after 5min if no better)	Adult	500 mcg = 0.5 mL
	Child > 12y	500 mcg = 0.5 mL
	Child 6-12y	300 mcg = 0.3 mL
	Child < 6y	150 mcg = 0.15 mL
Chlorphenamine IM	Adult or child > 12y	10 mg
	Child 6-12 y	5 mg
	Child 6m – 6y	2.5 mg
	Child < 6m	250 mcg/kg
Hydrocortisone IM	Adult or child > 12y	200 mg
	Child 6-12 y	100 mg
	Child 6m – 6y	50 mg
	Child < 6m	25 mg
IVF (Crystalloid)	Adult	500 – 1000 mL
	Child	20 mL/kg

- **Cardiac arrest in adults**
  - o 30:2 compressions to breaths (2 min cycle)
  - o Adrenaline given every 3-5 mins (every alternate CPR cycle)
  - o Amiodarone after 3 shocks
  - o Rhythm
    - ▪ Shockable (VF/pulseless VT) → 1 shock & resume CPR cycle
    - ▪ Non-shockable (PEA/asystole) → no shock, resume CPR cycle
  - o Treat reversible causes: 4 Hs (hypoxia, hypovolaemia, hypo/hyperkalaemia, hypothermia), 4 Ts (thrombosis, tension PTX, tamponde, toxins)

2. RESPIRATORY MEDICINE

GENERAL TIPS

- Common conditions are common – know asthma and COPD inside out.

- The NICE and BTS guidelines for asthma and COPD differs – we would use the NICE guidelines for this examination.

- Weird infections and occupational disease are favourite topics.

OBSTRUCTIVE LUNG CONDITIONS

- Obstructive conditions give rise to wheeziness. Coarse crackles on top of wheeze could indicate secondary infection or bronchiectasis.
- The spirometry findings for obstructive disease is FEV1/FVC < 0.7.

Asthma

- Diagnosis: asthma-COPD overlap

Increases probability of asthma	Lower probability of asthma
1. Main Sx =wheeze, SOB, chest tightness	**Prominent** dizziness, light-headedness, tingling
2. Diurnal **variation**	**Chronic** productive cough, with no wheeze
3. Response to exercise, allergen, cold air Seasonal or year-to-year variations, no progression	Sx with colds only Progressively worsens
4. Sx after **ASA** or BB	**Change in voice**
5. Hx atopy (or previous Dx asthma)	*Cardiac disease* (not all wheezes are asthma); previous Dx of COPD etc.
6. FHx atopy/asthma	**Smoking Hx significant (> 20 PY)**
7. Widespread wheeze (can be expiratory $\pm$ inspiratory) heard on auscultation	Normal examination when Sx
8. Unexplained low FEV1 or PEF <u>during</u> Sx (NORMAL in between Sx)	Normal PEF **during** Sx **Or in COPD = persistently abnormal between Sx**; post-bronchodilator challenge FEV1/FVC < 0.7
9. Unexplained **eosinophilia**	
10. Age onset < 20y	Age onset > 40 y
11. CXR normal	CXR shows lungs hyperinflated
12. Immediate response to bronchodilators (or response to steroids over weeks); may be self-limited	Rapid-acting bronchodilators only provide LIMITED relief.

- NICE says if high probability of asthma – Tx as asthma
- If intermediate probability – test for <u>bronchodilator reversibility</u> with spirometry (>15% improvement)
  - Other tests: eosinophilic inflammation (bloods; Fractiomal Exhaled NO = FeNO high e.g. > 40 ppb), atopy (IgE), methacholine challenge (not licensed and last resort if FeNO equivocal)
    - FeNO lowered by smoking.

- o Occupational asthma – worse during work. Remits when away from work (weekends or on holidays). Example: food processors, animal handlers, welders, paint sprayers. **Dx: peak flow diary** to assess trends.
- Asthma ladder for asthma (ascend or descend if >/<3X Sx per week respectively; proper inhaler technique – spacer to reduce static charge to deliver drug)
  - o Step 1: SABA PRN (good for exercise induced)
  - o Step 2: SABA PRN + low-dose ICS **maintenance**
  - o Step 3: ICS + SABA + LTRA
  - o Step 4: LABA + ICS (review LTRA)
  - o Step 5: MART (ICS + LABA) + LTRA
- Drugs:

Beta 2 agonists	Short-acting (SABA) – salbutamol. Works acutely. Long-acting (LABA) – salmeterol. DELAYED onset. Reduces *nocturnal Sx.* S/E: tachycardia, tremor/anxiety, cramps, *paradoxical bronchospasm* **Increases lactate** (false +ve on blood gas), **hypokalemia** (used as Tx of hyperkalaemia), **hyperglycaemia**
Steroids	Act over days. Can be inhaled (ICS) or oral/IV (acute for 5-7 days; chronic if still uncontrolled by ICS). Aimed to be at lowest dose Require bone and GI protection. May cause thrush (inhaled route – PPx: rinse mouth after usage). Long-term use may lead to adrenal suppression → steroid card: if patient is sick – may need doubling of dose to cover sick days. High acute dose can cause psychoses. May cause reactive leucocytosis (high WCC). But patients are "immunosuppressed".
MART = ICS+LABA	This helps with compliance.
Leukotriene receptor antagonists	PO montelukast Additive effect with ICS. S/E: abdo pain, thirst, headache. Very rare association with drug-induced Churg-Strauss syndrome (or may unmask Churg-SDtrauss) → eosinophilia, vasculitic rash, pulmonary-renal syndrome.
Aminophyllines	Theophylline (nocte to prevent morning dipping) – rarely used in primary care because: 1. Zero-order kinetics = saturable and metabolised by liver (variation in smokers, liver/heart failures) 2. Affected by inducers 3. Narrow therapeutic index – toxicity: GI upset (N), tachycardia (ECG monitoring), seizures, hypokalaemia, hyperglycaemia
Sodium cromoglicate	INH mast cell stabilisers **PPx in mild and exercise-induced asthma** esp. kiddos.
Anticholinergics	Short-acting (SAMA) – ipratropium

	Long-acting (LAMA) – tiotropium More used in COPD.
Omalizumab	Anti-IgE Mab used in persistent allergic asthma in secondary care
Mepolizumab	Anti-IL5 Mab used in refractory eosinophilic asthma in 2° care

Inhalers:

BLUE (SABA)	GREEN (LABA)	PURPLE (LABA)	BROWN (ICS)

- Acute exacerbation of asthma in **adults**
  - Moderate: PEF > 50-75%
    - TX: SABA nebulisers, PO prednisolone
  - Severe: (1) cannot form sentences, (2) HR > 110 bpm, (3) RR > 25/min, (4) PEFR **33-50%**.
    - Tx: admit. As above but additionally consider single dose IV magnesium if PEFR < 50%.
  - Life-threatening: (1) silent chest/confused/cyanosis, (2) HR **can be bradycardic**, (3) RR **can be low due to exhaustion** ($PaCO_2$ increasing is a worrying sign due to CO_2 retention from fatigue-related hypoventilation = near-fatal), (4) PEFR<33% predicted.
    - Tx: admit and likely need ventilatory support (intubation). Medical Tx as above **but add** SAMA.
    - Unlike COPD, you <u>do not NIV them</u>.
- Other features commonly tested:
  - Samter triad = asthma + nasal polyp + aspirin sensitivity
  - Beta blockers are contraindicated in severe asthma
  - Increased risk of developing pneumothorax – think of this when there is a very sudden onset of breathless out of proportion to the usual exacerbation

COPD (including NIV and LTOT stuff)
- Severity: GOLD categories
  - Mild: FEV1 $\geq$ 80%
  - Moderate: FEV1 50-79%
  - Severe: FEV1 30-49%
  - Very severe: FEV1 < 30%
- No clubbing!
- COPD ladder for chronic management
  - Step 1: SABA <u>or</u> SAMA
  - Step 2: LABA + LAMA if no asthmatic Sx or steroid responsiveness
    - If asthmatic features or steroid responsiveness: LABA + ICS
    - **Should not give steroids (ICS) alone – increase mortality as risk of pneumonia; *c.f.* combined LABA+ICS improve outcomes**
  - Step 3: 3-month trial of LABA + LAMA + ICS
    - If no improvement, revert back to LABA and LAMA.

Anti-	SAMA = ipratropium bromide; LAMA = tiotropium.

Muscarinics	**Indications:** LAMA is used in COPD; SAMA is used in asthma exacerbations. **Common S/E:** dry mouth (anti-M). **Less common S/E:** N + headache **Rare S/E:** constipation, tachycardia, retention*, confusion, blurred vision as dilated pupils, angle-closure glaucoma*; hypersensitivity. *****Caution:** BPH and glaucoma-prone patients **Interactions:** concomitant use of > 1 drug with anti-M (anti-cholinergic) effect increases risk of the toxidrome, esp. in **elderly** (however, inhaled meds rarely have such interactions).

Anti-cholinergic toxicity: Mad as hatter, blind as bat, full as flask, dry as bone, hot as hare, red as beet.

- Other Tx: annual flu + PC vaccine; pulmonary rehab (prevent muscle wasting and deconditioning); mucolytics
- Main prognostic improvement = STOP smoking. LTOT has some mortality benefit.

Long-term oxygen therapy
- Must not smoke (oxygen will explode) and
- PaO_2 < 7.3 persistently (2 values, > 3 weeks apart) despite maximum Tx; or
- PaO_2 < 8 and evidence of pulmonary hypertension (RVH, peripheral oedema), polycythaemia, or nocturnal hypoxia; or
- Palliative

- Exacerbation of COPD
  - NEB SAMA + SABA
  - Controlled O_2 (Venturi) – subgroup at risk of retention. Target sats 88-92%. **However, in patients who are acutely ill, they are at risk of dying from hypoxaemia – so high flow O_2 may be warranted.**
  - Steroids.
  - If infective exacerbation – add amoxicillin
  - If no response to above
    - IV aminophylline loading dose (ECG monitoring required)
    - Non-invasive ventilation:
      - RR > 30, **pH < 7.35**, $PaCO_2$ rising despite best medical care
    - Intubation:
      - **Jump to immediately if pH < 7.26**
      - Or when $PaCO_2$ rising despite NIV
  - Ensure no PTX

Cystic fibrosis

- Autosomal **recessive** (Ch7 CFTR gene); carrier rate 1:25 Caucasians
- All UK neonates are screened at birth (heel-prick at day 5 of life to look for immunoreactive trypsin, IRT)
    - High IRT suggest pancreatic injury but **non-specific** and may either need repeating in a few weeks **or nowadays** CFTR mutation PCR screen
    - Sweat test (ages 2y+) – **high Na + Cl** (defective NaCl CFTR channels)
    Neonatal presentation of CF – failure to thrive, meconium ileus, rectal prolapse
- Respiratory presentation of CF – recurrent chest infections, nasal polyps, eventually lead to bronchiectasis
- GI presentation of CF – pancreatic insufficiency = diabetes + steatorrhea; *distal intestinal obstruction* (adult version of meconium ileus), gallstones, cirrhosis
- Others – **male infertility** (undeveloped vas + epididymis); *female subfertility*; arthritis; clubbing; depression.
- Management is multifactorial:
    - Physiotherapy
    - Abx for acute infective exacerbation
        - *Staph aureus, Pseudomonas, Burkholderia cepacian*
        - Azithromycin is anti-inflammatory in nature
    - Mucolytics e.g. DNAse
    - Bronchodilators
    - Immunisation and yearly CXR surveillance
    - O_2/diuretics/NIV if cor pulmonale; *bilateral* lung-heart transplant (**contraindication for transplant** = *Burkholderia cepacia*).
    - Creon
    - Ursodeoxycholic acid for liver impairment; cirrhosis → liver transplant
    - Diabetic management (yearly OGTT from age 12)
    - Special drugs:
        - Ivacaftor (CFTR potentiator) for G551D mutation (leads to opening defects of channels) → potentiate gating of CFTR channels
        - Lumacaftor (CFTR corrector) for classic *F508Δ* mutation (leads to misprocessing of channel) → correct cell surface-localisation of channel proteins

Bronchiectasis

- **Permanent** airway dilatation and thinning → persistent cough and copious sputum +/- intermittent haemoptysis, constitutional symptoms with weight loss
- Causes: blockage, extrinsic narrowing, congenital*, infective, inflammation
    - *Young syndrome: obstructive azoospermia + chronic sino-pulmonary infections → bronchiectasis
    - *Primary ciliary dyskinesia e.g. Kartagener's syndrome – cilia fail in upper respiratory + hearing system; embryologically; and in reproductive system → respectively causes: paranasal sinusitis + bronchiectasis, hearing loss, situs inversus, and infertility
- CXR – tramline and ring shadows = thickened bronchial walls
- High-resolution CT scan → small airway dilatation more than nearby vessels (Signet ring sign = dilated bronchus with pulmonary artery nearby); cysts; mucous plugging

- Management includes: airway clearance (PT, mucolytics), bronchodilators, long-term antibiotics or preventive ones (can be *inhaled*; azithromycin is anti-inflammatory in nature), steroids, surgery if localised.

RESTRICTIVE LUNG CONDITIONS
- Restrictive conditions give rise to FINE crackles that do not change on inspiration/expiration, coughing, or movement. Associated w bronchial sounds.
- The spirometry findings for restrictive disease is $FEV1/FVC \geq 0.7$.

Interstitial lung diseases
- Diffuse chronic inflammation that is progressive.
- Presents as **dry cough**, **exertional SOB**, clubbing.
- Gold-standard Dx: **high-resolution CT scan (HRCT)**
- Classification and nomenclature change every few years and is not worth memorising
- Tx – steroids → cyclophosphamide if refractory +/- azathioprine.
- Key complication: **cor pulmonale** – right-sided heart failure (requires LTOT), and infections. 10X increased risk of lung cancer.

Sarcoidosis
- Multi-system granulomatous inflammation
  - Lungs: Stage 0 = no changes
    - Stage 1 = BHL
    - Stage 2 = BHL + peripheral pulmonary infiltrates
    - Stage 3 = solely peripheral pulmonary infiltrates
    - Stage 4 = progressive fibrosis, honeycombing (bullae), pleural
  - Endocrine – **hypercalcaemia, hypercalcuria** (renal stones)
  - Cardiomyopathy
  - ENT/Eyes – uveitis, sicca, parotid gland enlargement
  - Bone cyst
  - Hepatosplenomegaly
  - Neuropathies (e.g. Bell's)
  - Skin manifestation: erythema nodosum (painful red shin nodules), *lupus pernio* (purple-blue lesions on distal ends: ears, nose, fingers, toes), *subcut nodules*.
- Lofgren's syndrome = fever, erythema nodosum, polyarthralgia **esp. ANKLES**, and bilateral hilar lymphadenopathy
- Labs: **hyeprcalcaemia** (giant cells in granuloma contain 1-alpha-hydroxylase), high serum ACE (non-specific), lymphopenia, high ESR
- Tx: **steroid course** +/- NSAIDs

Predilection of location of fibrosis

Apical fibrosis	Basal fibrosis
BREAST PX	*RACIST*
Bronchopulmonary aspergillosis	Rheumatoid arthritis
Radiotherapy	Asbestosis
EAA	Connective tissue disease/Cryptogenic
Ankylosing spondylosis	fibrosing alveolitis
Sarcoidosis	Idiopathic pulmonary fibrosis (usual)
TB	Scleroderma
Pneumoconiosis (coal worker's, etc.)	Treatments (drugs: bulsuphan, bleomycin,
Histiocytosis X	nitrofurantoin, hydralazine, MTX, amiodarone)

OCCUPATIONAL LUNG DISEASES

Asbestosis	ILD/ cancer	Fire-proofing, wire, pipe materials in olden days. *Amphibole* asbestos confer higher risk of mesothelioma versus "coloured" asbestos (e.g. most common: *chrysotile = white*). **More commonly leads to bronchial adenocarcinoma** rather than mesothelioma.
Berylliosis	ILD	Aerospace or nuclear industries
Silicosis	ILD	Pottery, sandblasting, quarrying (clay).
Coal worker's lung	ILD	Coal dust. Numerous small nodules. Black sputum/lung.
Caplan's disease		Coal worker's lung + rheumatoid arthritis + pulmonary rheumatoid nodules (cavities)
Malt worker's lung Farmer's lung Mushroom worker Sugar worker Bird Fancier	EAA	*Aspergillus clavatus* *Saccharopolyspora rectivirgula; actinomyces; micropolyspora* Thermophilic *Actinomyces* *Thermoactinomyces sacchari* Avian antigens

- Entitled to compensation

PULMONARY INFECTIONS

- CURB-65 score for severity of community acquired pneumonia:
  - Confusion (AMTS $\leq$ 8), Urea > 6, RR $\geq$ 30, **BP**: either systolic < 90 or diastolic < 60 mmHg
  - Score 0-1: low mortality – can discharge; score 2 – admit for IV Abx
- Atypical pneumonia – "walking pneumonia": insidious. Pt: malaise, headache, myalgia, arthalgia, dry-ish cough.

Characteristics of different pathogens in pneumonia

Bugs	Features	Dx/Tx
Strep pneumoniae	Most common. Weird presentations: herpes labialis	Urinary antigen CXR (lobar consolidation) Amoxicillin (penicillins)
Staph aureus	May complicate *flu* infection. IV drug users.	Flucloxacillin (Vancomycin if MSRA; linezolid/clindamycin if Panton-Valentine leucocidin = PVL) CXR (bilateral cavitations or patchiness)
Klebsiella	Elderly, diabetic, alcoholic Redcurrant sputum	CXR (cavitating upper lobe) Usually drug-resistant
ASPIRATION	Patients with unsafe swallows Anaerobes = foul sputum	May need to add gram negative/anaerobe cover e.g. metronidazole
Legionella	Atypical PNA. Thrive in water system e.g. air conditioners, cruise ships. **Hyponatraemia**, confusion, D/V, deranged LFTs, AKI, and lymphopenia	Urinary antigen CXR (bibasal consolidation) Macrolides or fluroquinolones
Mycoplasma	Atypical PNA. Winter epidemics. *Erythema multiforme* (target rash); **cold agglutinin** (IgM haemolytic anaemia in the cold); myocarditis; glomerulonephritis; meningoencephalitis.	Macrolides (as no cell wall – so penicillin just do not work) Fluroquinolones Tetracyclines
Chlamydia psittaci	Atypical PNA. Infected birds (parrots). Meningo-encephalitis, culture negative infective endocarditis, hepatitis, AKI, splenomegaly	Serology Tetracyclines Macrolides
Pseudomonas	Bronchiectasis and cystic fibrosis. Hospital-acquired (ITU) – tubes… Green sputum	Limited antibiotics work: Tazocin, ciprofloxacin, meropenem, gentamicin, ceftazidime
PCP	Immunosuppressed. Shortness of breath on exertion with low PaO_2.	CXR (ground glass opacification – bilateral perihilar interstitial shadowing) BAL Co-trimoxazole
TB	1. Pyrexia, night sweats, malaise, anorexia, clubbing, haemoptysis	Dx of latent TB – IGRA. Active TB is **notifiable**.

	and cough. **2. Cardio:** pericarditis **3. CNS/spine:** Pott's disease -> vertebral collapse (kyphoscoliosis, spinal compression); meningitis **4. GI & GU:** colicky abdo pain, loin pain, sterile pyuria and haematuria. **5. Derm:** erythema nodosum, lupus vulgaris (red-brown apple- jelly nodule). **6. Miliary:** disseminated by blood	Offer HIV testing PPx: BCG • High-risk (area with high TB, ≥ 1 parents/grandparents born in country with widespread TB, family with TB in past 5 years) neonates • Children ≤ 15 who are vaccinated as newborn and high-risk • Adults ≤ 35, negative Mantoux test, high-risk (close contact w TB, areas with widespread TB, animal work = chimpanzees/ cows, prisons/ residential home/ asylum seekers, going to country with widespread TB > 3m) • HIV **R**ifampicin – *inducer*, orange red urine and tears, transient hepatitis **I**soniazid – peripheral neuropathy (prophylactic pyridoxine = vitamin B6 replacement), hepatitis, drug-induced lupus. **P**yrazinamide – hepatitis, rash, arthralgia. Good meningeal penetration. Can ppt gout. **E**thambutol – red-green colour blindness, nystagmus and optic neuritis; peripheral neuropathy. **Steroids:** used in TB pericarditis/meningitis
Fungal	Immunosuppressed. **Aspergillus*.** **Candida:** ICU patient **Histoplasmosis:** bats (caves); birds **Blastomycosis:** compost (USA) **Cryptococcus:** pigeon droppings	Aspergillus serology. Cultures + PCR. Urine Ag, serology. KOH culture India ink stain and serology (CSF)
Viral pneumonia (Tx: supportive)	Influenza (annual flu jabs for vulnerables: >50y, pregnant, HCW, comorbid: diabetics, cardiovascular – not solely hypertension, respiratory etc.) • Complicated flu: **oseltamivir** (neuraminidase inhibitor) + O_2 • Post-exposure PPx: high risk <u>and</u> not protected by vaccine → **oseltamivir**. Swine flu (H1N1) – **zanamivir** used instead (oseltamivir resistance) Bird flu (avoid touching dead infected birds and their droppings/bedding) • Antiviral given 7-10 days after known exposure or 2 d of Sx onset. • Human-to-human transmission *not* possible.	

Aspergillus affects lung in 5 ways:
1. Asthma (type 1 hypersensitivity). **Tx: bronchodilators**

2. Allergic bronchopulmonary aspergillosis (type 1 and 3 hypersensitivity) – IgE RAST +ve, eosinophilia, raised IgE. **Tx: steroids.**

3. Extrinsic allergic alveolitis (EAA) – pneumonitis (type 3 and 4 hypersensitivity) from repeated exposure to spores (*Aspergillus clavatus* in **Malt worker's lung: barley**) → 4-6 hours post-exposure atypical pneumonia then chronically restrictive lung disease. **Tx: avoid exposure, oxygen, steroids.**

4. Aspergilloma. CXR: fungus ball in pre-existing lung cavity. **Tx: excision e.g. if massive haemoptysis; oral anti-fungals poor penetration.**

5. Invasive aspergillosis. Sick patient with weak immunity. Beta-glucan, serology and imaging. **Tx: azoles + amphotericin.**

LUNG CANCER

Characteristics of different types of lung cancer
- Non-small cell carcinoma – Tx: surgery

Small (oat) cell lung CA	Smokers	SIADH (hyponatraemia) Cushing's syndrome (ectopic ACTH) Lambert-Eaton syndrome (weakness relieved by exertion due to anti-voltage gated calcium channels) **Chemoradio-sensitive ("too SMALL for surgery")**
Squamous cell CA		Central. PTH-related protein (hypercalcaemia)
Adenocarcinoma	Non-smoker. Females. < 45y. Hypertrophic osteoarthropathy.	Peripheral. KRAS, EGFR, ALK mutations. No characteristic paraneoplastic
Large cell CA	Highly anaplastic	Peripheral. No characteristic paraneoplastic
Carcinoid	Carcinoid syndrome – flushing, diarrhoea, wheeze (5-HT)	
Mets	Cannonball mets – primary: RCC. MCC – breast anc colon carcinoma	
Pancoast tumour	Horner's syndrome: ipsilateral ptosis, miosis, anhidrosis	
Mesothelioma	Pleural cell tumour encasing the lung. No aetiological relation to smoking. Recurrent pleural effusions and pleurisy. Chemo-sensitive; pleurodesis and drainage. Poor prognosis.	

Solitary pulmonary nodule
- Factors favouring cancer (Brook's model) – female, older, FHx, larger, emphysema, upper lobe, low nodule sub-solid, spiculated
- < 5mm nodules (non-calcified) can be discharged
- If no previous imaging – CT scan e.g. in 3 months to assess growth
- If stable over 2 years, can generally discharge

PULMONARY EMBOLISM

- Risk factors: Embolic Hx, Baby, Oestrogen, Large, Immobile, Surgery, Malignancy
- Well's score ($\geq$ 4 = likely): "Don't Die, Tell Team To Calculate Criteria"
  - DVT Sx **+3**
  - Dx likely PE **+3**
  - Tachycardia **+1.5**
  - > Three days immobilisation/ Thirty days of surgery **+1.5**
  - Thromboembolism in past **+1.5**
  - Coughing up blood (haemoptysis) **+1**
  - Cancer (active Tx, in past 6 months, or palliative) **+1**
- **Investigations:**
  - D-dimer (not specific, *after 50 years old:* normal upper limit is usually 10 x age). A negative D-dimer rule OUT PE (high sensitivity).
  - **Gold-standard is CTPA** (RCOG has recommended this even in pregnant ladies!)
  - V:Q scan if CTPA absolutely contraindicated (renal impairment, contrast allergy)
  - Lower limb ultrasound if DVT suspected.
- Management:
  - Consider fluids
  - Treatment-dose low-molecular weight heparin (unfractionated if renally impaired) for 5 days
  - Bridge to warfarin (Stop LMWH when INR > 2; aim 2-3) or DOAC
  - Thrombolysis (with alteplase) is only used if haemodynamically unstable, with evidence of right heart strain. **Contraindicated if:** recent bleeding, recent high-risk events (spinal surgery, major trauma etc.), known history of stroke esp. haemorrhagic, uncontrolled hypertension, or severe liver disease.
  - Vena cava filter if anticoagulation is contraindicated.
- Unprovoked PE – **find an underlying cancer.** Anticoagulation $\geq$ 3-6 months to lifelong.
- Provoked PE – anticoagulation 3 months.

PLEURAL EFFUSIONS

- Light's criteria can be used to determine if a fluid is exudative, when the protein contain between 2.5 – 3.5 g/dL

Exudate (>3 – 3.5 g/dL)	Transudate (<2.5 g/dL)
Inflammations and infections: empyema, parapneumonic, TB, cancers	3 failures: heart, liver, renal Hypothyroidism. Meig's syndrome (unilateral transudate (usually right) with ascites and ovarian fibroma).
Effusion protein/serum protein > 0.5	< 0.5
Effusion LDH/serum LDH > 0.6	< 0.6
Effusion LDH > 2/3 upper limit normal	< 2/3

- **Appearances:** exudate and transudate are straw-coloured; turbid & yellow effusions are infective; blood can indicate trauma, cancer, or infarction.
- **Cytology:** neutrophils imply acute infection; lymphocytes imply chronic disease; RA has multinucleated gfiant cells.
- **Bacteriology:** ADA is increased in TB but also rheumatoid effusions (check for RhF)

PNEUMOTHORAX

- Primary pneumothorax
  - SOB ± rim of air > 2 cm → aspirate → if fail: chest drain
  - ASx ± rim of air < 2 cm → discharge and review in 1 month
- Secondary pneumothorax
  - SOB ± rim of air > 2 cm → chest drain
  - If ASx and size 1-2cm → aspirate + admit to observe for 24 hours (CXR)
  - If ASx and < 1 cm → admit to observe for 24 hours (CXR)
- Size of PTX is measured from 1st visible lung margin to chest wall at level of hilum.
- **Tension pneumothorax** (haemodynamically compromised, trachea sucked TO side of lesion, hyperresonance) should be immediately relieved by **NEEDLE thoracocentesis.**
- Surgical treatment if bilateral pneumothoraces; failure of lung expansion 2 days after drain; 3rd episode same side; previous contralateral PTX

OBESITY AND LUNGS
- Obesity hypoventilation syndrome – daytime hypercapnia with or without actual airway obstruction.
- OSA – worsen by alcohol, smoking. Other than daytime sleepiness (measured by Epworth score) and cognitive effect, can also cause decreased libido. Tx: lifestyle advice, sleeping and positioning technique, routine referral for assessment – may need nocturnal CPAP.

ADJUNCT AIRWAYS
- Oropharyngeal airway – measured from incisor to angle of jaw. Used if *no* cough and gag reflex; otherwise may cause laryngospasm and vomiting from gag reflex stimulation.
- Nasopharyngeal airway – sized using internal diameter: size 6 for females, and size 7 for males generally. If cough and gag reflex intact. May be used in **seizing** patients (to avoid oral trauma or if mouth is tightly spastic). **Contraindicated** in facial trauma and base of skull fractures.
- Laryngeal mask airway – if BVM unsuccessful at restoring oxygenation despite above 2 adjuncts.
- Surgical airway e.g. tracheostomy. Last resort when LMA fails.

3. NEPHROLOGY

> **GENERAL TIPS**
> - Common renal issues are common – do not dwell too much on the subtypes of nephrotic and nephritic syndromes
>
> - You should memorise nephrotoxic medications and prescribing in CKD.

ACUTE KIDNEY INJURY
- Potentially reversible fast decline, KDIGO 2012 measured by <u>creatinine</u> and <u>urine output</u>
- Presentation <u>uraemia</u>, <u>acidosis</u>, <u>hyperkalaemia</u>, <u>fluid overload</u>
- At risk in old patients, volume depletion, cardiac insufficiency, antihypertensives (especially ACEi/ARB), iodine contrast, systemic illness (diabetes/myeloma)

Pre-renal (66%)	Volume depletion	Haemorrhage, gut loss, dehydration, burns, diuretics, DKA
Measure BP,	Systemic vasodilation	Sepsis, anti HTN, anaphylaxis
volume status *If don't treat*	Intrarenal vasoconstriction	AA/dissection, renal artery stenosis (FMD) NSAIDs, ACEi, tacrolimus, aminoglycosides
→ ATN, takes *6-8w recover*	Fluid redistribution	Hepatorenal, cardiorenal, cardiac pump failure (MI, arrhythmias, valve, tamponade, PE)
Renal (20%)	Glomerular	GPA/SLE, Anti GBM, post-strep
Urine dip,	Interstitial (polyuria first)	**TIN:** NSAIDs, PPI, cephalosporins, penicillin, strep, EBV/CMV/HIV, sarcoid, allergic
Stop *nephrotoxic* *agents*	Tubules	Ischaemia (**ATN**), toxins (radiocontrast, amoglycosides, cisplatin), tumour lysis, MTX, cisplatin, rhabdomyolysis, AIN (hypersensitivity)
	Vascular	RV thrombosis, scleroderma, atheroembolic disease, shock, HUS, TTP, vasculitis
Post renal *USS + bladder*	Intrarenal	Light chain precipitation, urate sludge – tumour lysis, oxalate – ethylene glycol
o/e and *catheter*	Bilateral tract	Stones, retroperitoneal fibrosis, papillary necrosis (analgesia, pyelonephritis, sickle)
	Urethral obstruction	Posterior valve, retroperitoneal fibrosis, BPH, prostate cancer, urethral strictures
	Others	Tb, post-op, neuropathy

- Acute vs chronic – chronic high creatinine and well, low calcium, high phosphate, high PTH, high ALP, abnormal bones, low Hb (<u>except PKD protected against anaemia</u>), USS kidney small (<u>unless early diabetes, amyloid, PKD, HIVAN, hydronephrosis</u>)

- Imaging kidneys – USS first choice, CTKUB (no contrast, pick up stones), CTU (contrast, not effective if eGFR low)
- Pre-renal vs ATN
  - Pre-renal: urine <u>less sodium, osmolality high, less urea excreted</u> (can concentrate)
  - ATN: urine <u>more sodium, osmolality same as plasma (low), see casts</u>
- Manage – ABCDE, <u>Stop DAMN</u> (diuretics, ACEi/ARB, metformin, NSAIDs), treat <u>reversible cause</u> (shock: fluid challenge, obstruction: image for cause & urology, urosepsis: sepsis 6), monitor <u>urine output (catheterise)/fluid balance/weight</u>
- Dialysis if (AEIOU)
  - Acidosis (pH <7.2)
  - Electrolytes (refractory K+ >6.5)
  - Intoxication (poisoning e.g. aspirin)
  - Oedema (pulmonary)
  - Uraemia (encephalopathy, pericarditis)

<u>Intrinsic renal disease</u>
- <u>Glomerular</u> – nephrotic/nephritic vs <u>tubulointerstitial</u> – TIN (tubulointerstitial nephritis), renal tubular acidosis, hereditary tubular diseases, polycystic kidney disease

<u>Nephrotic syndrome</u>
- Proteinuria (>3.5g/d), Hypoalbuminaemia (<30g/dl), Oedema
- Present: polyuria, polydipsia, frothy urine, oliguria, anuria, breathlessness, fatigue
- Associated: <u>Hyperlipidaemia</u> (lipid profile, lipiduria → IHD), <u>Hypercoagulability</u> (VTE – lose antithrombin III), <u>Infection</u> (low Ig, low C'), <u>Hypocalcaemia</u> (vitamin D and binding protein lost in urine)
- Management: All Na+ & fluid restrict, diuretics, LMWH, <u>trial steroids</u> (90% relapse children), if no response to steroids: <u>biopsy</u>
- Histopathology
  - Minimal change – Hodgkin's, NSAIDs, young, fused podocytes, 2/3 recur, treatment <u>steroids (80% respond) → cyclophosphamide if resistant</u>, outcome: 1/3 one episode, 1/3 infrequent relapse, 1/3 frequent relapse
  - Membraneous – idiopathic (<u>antiphospholipase A2</u>), cancer 5-10% (prostate/lung/lymphoma/leukaemia) gold/penicillamine/NSAID, hep B/malaria/syphilis/HIV, rx <u>ACEi/ARB</u>, if progressive <u>combination steroid + cyclophosphamide</u>
  - FSGS – young adults, 1o (most common idiopathic) or 2o: <u>DM</u>, amyloid, collapsing (<u>heroin</u>/HIV), obesity, sickle– knock out some glomeruli, Alport), IgM deposition, rx steroids/cyclophos, high in transplants, 50% → ESRF
  - Diabetic - 1 hyperfiltration (increase GFR), 2 silent/latent (GFR increase, most don't progress for 10 years), 3 incipient (microalbuminuria 30-300/d), 4 overt (persistent proteinuria >300mg/d, dipstick positive, HTN, bx Kimmelstiel-Wilson nodules diffuse glomerulosclerosis and focal glomerulosclerosis), 5 end stage (GFR <10)
  - Amyloid – AL myeloma/Waldenstrom/MGUS, AA – TB/bronchiectasis/RA/JIA

- ○ **SLE** (check ANA/DNA binding) – diffuse proliferative

Nephritic syndrome
- Haematuria, Reduced GFR (oliguria, <u>uraemia</u>, fluid retention), Hypertension (headache, LVH)
- Cause proliferative vs cresenteric
- **IgA** – 3-5% pop, most asymptomatic, synphayngeal (1-2d after URTI), associated coeliac, young, male, macroscopic haematuria, 25% ESRF, worse if HTN, smoking, hyperlipidaemia, male
- **HUS** – kids, acute renal failure, MAHA, thrombocytopenia, e. coli 0157:H7 (Shiga toxin), tumours, pregnancy, ciclosporin, OCP, SLE, HIV, **Ix** – FBC, U&E, stool, **Management** – supportive (fluids, transfusion, dialysis), no Abx
- **Rapidly progressive GN (cresenteric)**
    - ○ <u>Goodpastures</u> (HLA-DR2, men, bimodal (20/60), IgG basement membrane, rx plasma exchange, steroids, cyclophosphamide, % pulmonary haemorrhage – smoking, LRTI, pulmonary oedema, inhale hydrocarbon, young male
    - ○ **ANCA positive GPA/MPA/EGPA**

Both nephrotic and nephritic
- **Membranoproliferative glomerulonephritis** – 50% will have ESRF, 3 types, 1 (90%) <u>cryoglobulinaemia, hep C</u>, 2 <u>partial lipodystrophy/factor H deficiency</u>, 3 <u>hep B/C</u>
- **Diffuse proliferative glomerulonephritis** – post strep GN (check ASOT, low C'3 (IgG IgM and C3 deposition), **SLE lupus type IV**

Tubulointerstitial nephritis
- Can't concentrate (polyuria/nocturia/thirst/glycosuria), can't reabsorb (glucose/Pi/AA appearing urine), <u>allergic</u> to drugs/infection (WCC, eosinophils), urticaria + fever + arthralgia
- Causes <u>drugs</u> (NSAIDs, Abx – ceph, <u>penicillin</u>, <u>rifampicin</u>, sulphonamide, diuretics – <u>frusemide</u>, thiazide, <u>allopurinol</u>, cimetidin), infections (staph, strep, CMV/EBV/toxo, Hanta), immune (sarcoid, Sjogren's), *chronic TIN fibrosis caused by reflux/chronic pyelonephritis, DM, SCD or trait*
- <u>Cf AIN</u> – TIN is inflammatory, so higher WCC
- <u>Rx:</u> Stop offending drug, fluids, prednisolone

Renal tubular acidosis
- Distal (can't excrete H+), <u>bad</u>, Marfan's, ED, Sjogren's = less K+
- Proximal (reabsorb bicarb), Fanconi = less K+, from cytinosis, Sjogren, myeloma, nephrotic syndrome, Wilson's. Present: polyuria, in urine: amino/glycol/phosphate, osteomalacia
- Resistance or deficiency, older = high K+

Hereditary tubular conditions
- Bartter's – block NaKCC in loop (like furosemide) – metabolic alkalosis
- Gitelman – block NaCl in DCT (like thiazide) – metabolic alkalosis, hypocalciuria

ADULT POLYCYSTIC KIDNEY DISEASE

- Type 1 chromosome 16 (80%), type 2 chromosome 4
- Loin pain, palpable kidneys, gross haematuria following trauma, UTI, stones, polyuria + nocturia, haemorrhage and infected into cyst, 70% ESRF by 70y
- **Extrarenal**: **HTN**, infertility (seminal vesicles), 70% liver cysts, 25% **mitral valve prolapse**/aortic root dilation, aortic dissection, MR/TR, 8% berry → SAH, cysts in pancreas, spleen, (rarely: thyroid, oesophagus, ovary)
- Image USS/CT, diagnose if FHx+ve and 2 cysts (<30y), 2 both kidneys (30-59), 4 both (>60)
- Rx - **General:** Drink more, less salt and caffeine, monitor U&E and BP, avoid contact sports, genetic counselling, MRA screen for berry aneurysms, **medical:** statin/aspirin, HTN (<130/80 with ACEi), treat infections, **surgical:** laparoscopic cyst removal, nephrectomy, **50% ESRF:** dialysis or transplant by age 60yo
- C.f. **Autosomal recessive PKD** 1/40,000, infancy, renal cysts, hepatic fibrosis

CHRONIC KIDNEY DISEASE

- eGFR measures (falls with age) + proteinuria, needs 2 values at **3mo** (staging system not diagnosis), only diagnose 1 and 2 if supported by evidence (urinalysis or renal mass)

1. >90 – normal, but can still have kidney disease (proteinuria)
2. 60-90 – falls with age, so need kidney damage
3. 30-59 – a (above 45), b (below 45)
4. 15-29
5. <15

- Slow progression with BUPA: **B**lood pressure + proteinuria (**130/80** <1g/d or DM, **125/75** if higher), Rx first line **ACEi** (CI – fixed stenosis upstream, pregnancy oligohydramnios, prev hypersensitivity/angioedema), repeat U&Es – **1w after starting** pick up hyperkalaemia, disproportionate rise in creatinine for renal artery stenosis, **U**nderlying illness (DM control), **P**rotein intake (avoid K+, Pi), **A**void obstruction/dehydration/infection/nephrotoxics

Complications of CKD ("A to L"):

- Anaemia
    - Decreased erythropoiesis: EPO interstitium once **eGFR <30**, consider other causes if eGFR is >60, in blood loss e.g., capillary fragility, poor platelet function, stress ulceration, aluminium toxic (it's rare now cos we monitor), functional Fe deficiency e.g. inappropriate high hepcidin from kidneys, shortened RBC survival e.g. haemodialysis, parathyroid disease, uraemia inhibit BM, intercurrent inflammation (ACD))
    - Predisposes to development of LV hypertrophy
    - Check haemotyinics, TFTs, myeloma, optimise iron status before EPO

- o   Give **Fe²⁺ IV (**dextran) + **EPO** (eprex 1-3/week **s/c**: is peptide hormone but when dialysing can give **IV through machine)**
- o   Raise Hb to **11g/dL** (higher – thrombosis risk)
- Bones (skeleton – pain, fractures, deformity, ostitis fibrosa, osteomalacia, adynamic bone, calcium – itch, soft tissue calcification, skin necrosis, red eyes, muscles – proximal myopathy)
  - o   XR – brown tumour, Looser's zone, rugger jersey spine over long time (chronicity)
  - o   Pathology:
    - **Less active vitamin D (**less 1a-OH vit D) → less inhibition PTH
    - **More plasma Pi (less excretion)**, decreased plasma Ca2+ → higher PTH (2ⁿᵈ) → bone breakdown (more ALP, release Ca2+ and Pi) → over time 3ʳᵈ autonomous
  - o   Give **1α calcidiol, less Pi diet, Pi binders** (calcium acetate, carbonate – also increase Ca²⁺), **remove parathyroid** (surgery), **calcimimetic** (cinacalcet)
- CVD (calcification, also anaemia, malnutrition, risk factors like HTN, CCF, DM)
  - o   **Rx statins, low-dose, lifestyle, BP control**
- Drug-related side effects
- Emotions (including sexual dysfunction)
- Fluid (pulmonary oedema) → IV furosemide
- Growth
- Hypertension
- Immunosuppression → immunise influenza and pneumococcus
- Joints
- Killed by kidneys (death)
- Legs restless → *clonazepam*

Renal replacement therapy

HD	PD	RT
3 treatments, 3-5h, access, (hosp/satellite/home) AVF (radial artery + cephalic vein) or tesio	CAPD: 4/d, 3-4h, 8h overnight APD: 8-20L, 8h overnight 4-6 clinic visits (home, self/carer) Tenckhoff catheter 2-3w before	Check virology (CMV, HCV, HBV, HIV, VZV, EBV), CVD, TB, ABO + HLA, psych assess, in HBD and NHBD, living (10%) better prognosis
Profession provides care Regular review	Better in first 2y (preserve renal function), if haemodynamic unstable, bad veins, flexible, no diet restriction or needles	Best prognosis (95% survival 1y, 90% graft survival), 15y graft survival, DM can pancreas + kidney Cheaper long term
Neg: Need travel, fixed schedule, permanent internal access, 2 needle sticks, diet + fluid restrict (avoid high K+), haemodynamic instability from fluid removal, arrhythmia AVF: 6-8w mature, infection, thrombosis, steal syndrome, stenosis	**CI**: major abdo sx (adhesions), poor motivation, hygiene, emaciation, COPD, -ostomy **Neg:** Infection and blockage (staph epidermis), PD peritonitis (send fluid for WCC, MCS, gram stain – see strip), not long term (2-5y), membrane failure, fibrosis, sclerosis, long term damage to peritoneum, weight gain (fluid, glucose), back pain, malnutrition, supplies at home	**CI:** 30% not suitable (below) **Neg:** Frequent clinic visits early, DVT/PE, immunosuppression (tumour, infection), recurrent disease, drug toxicity, CV risk persists, graft failure
Sepsis, blood loss, IE, disequilibriation syndrome, bioincompatibility	Encapsulating peritoneal sclerosis (rare), hernia	Bleeding, graft thrombosis, infection, leaks, rejection

- Based on patient preference
- Conservative – preserve renal function with BUPA, minimise symptoms
- **Diseases may recur in transplant:** primary GN (MPGN mainly), Goodpasture, familial HUS, diabetes, hyperoxaluria, **Alport post-transplant** (developed AutoAb to *normal* collagen IV that the body "has never seen before" due to inherited defect → Goodpasture's syndrome of the transplanted kidney)
- **Rejection** - Match HLA (on chromosome 6) DR > B> A
  - Hyperacute (m/hr) – type II hypersensitivity IgG → vessel thrombosis, from Ab vs ABO/HLA
  - Acute (<6mo) – mismatched HLA/CMV, cytotoxic T-cell mediated, rx steroid/imunosuppress
  - Chronic (>6mo) – Ab and cell fibrosis to kidney (chronic allograft nephropathy) or recurrence (MCGN > IgA > FSGS)

Prescribing in CKD

- **Excreted/metabolism (don't change loading, reduce maintenance dose):**
Reduce opiates and digoxin, Stop metformin (MALA), Reduce glicazide/insulin
(hypos), Reduce LMWH and monitor activity, Reduce methotrexate

- **Increasing:** Diuretics – block tubular function, in renal they have less to work on,
also binds to albumin (furosemide), but beware of potassium sparing and over-
diuresis: If overloaded increase dose, underloaded stop, Stop spironolactone
(careful with K+), Thiazide → loop in CKD4-5, bb ok (liver) except atenolol and
bisoprolol, *Nitrofurantoin – stop at <60ml/min (useless)

- **Affect renal** Aminoglycoside antibiotics – drug monitoring, nephrotoxic but if no
other possible Abx then do have to use for infection, Tetracycline – stop unless
doxycycline (in CKD4-5), NSAIDs – if out of pain etc might be ok if mild CRF, on
dialysis, stop prostaglandin, can cause TIN, minimal change disease, Can change
to paracetamol, ACEi – if dehydration/RA stenosis/sepsis (over 24h), otherwise
protective, decrease in eGFR 25% or creatinine 30% is acceptable, Aspirin –
nephrotoxic, anticoagulant, but can keep at low cardioprotective, Lithium - stop

Potassium disorders
- Hypokalaemia
  - Work-up:
    - Step 0 – dangerous level: < 2.5 mmol/L → treat
    - Step 1 – Hx + low K+ → check **aldosterone: renin ratio** (if high = Conn's)
    - Step 2 – check **urinary K+** (if > 20 = **renal** cause e.g. Conn's, Cushing, Liddle's = ENac mutation, liquorice!!)
    - Step 3 – is there HTN? (No = **normotensive hypoK+** suggests *Bartter or Gitelman or renal tubular acidosis **type 1 or 2***).
      N.B. type 4 RTA leads to HYPERkalaemia
  - **Causes:**
    - Reduced intake
    - Excessive losses
      - Sweating; GI (including stoma!)
      - Endocrine (Cushing's, Conn's)
      - Renal (loop/thiazide, Bartter/Gitelman, RTA1/2, diuretics)
    - Transcellular shifts e.g. **alkalosis, salbutamol, insulin**, and rapid cell proliferation (cancer)
  - Presentation: cramps, tetany, weakness + palpitations (arrhythmias – ECG see *Cardiology*), **causes nephrogenic DI.**
  - Tx:
    - Mild – Sando K, K+ sparing diuretics
    - Severe – IV K
    - Replete magnesium (uncorrected Mg2+ cause refractory hypokalaemia)
- Hyperkalaemia
  - Causes: excess intake (TPN, antibiotics containing K+, K+ fluids, massive blood transfusion); reduced loss (Addison's, ACE-I, spironolactone, amiloride, **AKI**); transcellular shift (acidosis, tumour lysis, haemoylsis, rhabdomyolysis, beta blockers).
  - Pseudo-hyperkalaemia = haemolysis of blood sample
  - Pt: palpitations
  - Tx:
    - **Stop nephrotoxics**
    - Stabilisation of cardiac membranes with calcium gluconate
    - Salbutamol NEBs & 50 ml 50% IV dextrose with 10 units of insulin
    - PO/PR resin (calcium resonium) – only non-invasive way to deplete K+ (other methods cause transcellular shift): K+ loss through gut... but take days.
    - **Haemodialysis:** very high K+ > 7 or refractory

Acid-base balance

Step 1 – check pH
Step 2 – check HCO_3^- and PCO_2 to find culprit of change
Step 3 – for **metabolic acidosis ONLY**: calculate the **anion gap**
Step 4 – check for compensations (opposing the change)
Step 5 – check for **mixed disorders** (compensation exaggerated or very inadequate).

- Respiratory alkalosis
  - $PaCO_2$ **low** + pH > 7.45 $\pm$ renal compensation (**bicarb low**)
  - Causes:
    - Hyperventilation (anxiety MCC, pain, high altitude, ASA overdose*)
      a) High altitudes: low P_{ATM} → low P_{O2} → hyperventilation → low P_{CO2} → pH rise → over 23h, kidneys excrete bicarb and hyperventilation falls; use of acetazolamide augments bicarb excretion
      b) Aspirin overdose*: **mixed acid-base disorder**
        - Shortly after ingestion – salicylates stimulate medulla → hyperventilation
        - Hours later → produce **anion gap** metabolic acidosis → salicylic <u>acid</u> inhibits TCA cycles = increase pyruvate & stimulate lipolysis (fatty <u>acid</u> + keto<u>acids</u> increase) + uncouple OXPHOS (lactic <u>acid</u> increases)
        - Features: variable pH, low P_{CO2}
    - Restrictive lung diseases including sarcoidosis
    - Acute respiratory problem

- **Metabolic alkalosis**
  - **Bicarb high** + pH > 7.45 $\pm$ respiratory compensation ($PaCO_2$ **high**)
  - Causes:
    - **Contraction** alkalosis
      a) Reduce EBV → RAAS activation → AT-II → *H+ secretion* in proximal tubule and HCO_3^- reabsorption & **aldosterone** → *H+ secretion* to gain Na+ (intercalated cells of collecting duct)
      b) Example: **hyperaldosteronism** –contraction alkalosis of aldosterone
    - Vomiting – loses HCl and volume (contraction alkalosis). HCl loss → HCO3 generation (for every H+ generated, 1 bicarbonate left in blood); further more K+ is lost during vomiting = transcellular shift → alkalosis.
      a) **Urinary Cl is low in vomiting – good to spot surreptitious vomiting e.g. bulimia**
    - Hypokalaemia (transcellular shift)

- Diuretics
    a) Loops and thiazides
        - Leads to contraction alkalosis
        - Leads to hypokalaemia (transcellular shift)
        - Leads to increased sodium load and water delivery to distal nephron = more K+/H+ echanged for Na+ reabsorption
    b) Bartter syn (mimics loop) – NKCC defect of ascending limb
    c) Gitelman syn (mimics thiazide) – Na/Cl cotransporter defect of distal tubule
    d) **Surreptitious use of diuretics** to lose weight or reduce oedema (cosmetic) – initially increase urine clearance (inhibit Na & Cl reabsorption = water follows).
- Base ingestion e.g. antacids (milk-alkali syndrome, in the past) – antacids = Ca2+ and bicarb consumed → high Ca2+ **inhibiting NKCC** (TAL) and free **ADH**-dependent water absorption (hypercalcaemia causes NDI). Furthermore, antacid is an alkali base itself.

- Respiratory acidosis
    - $PaCO_2$ **high** + pH < 7.35 $\pm$ renal compensation (bicarb **high**)
    - Dangerous levels of acidosis is **< 7.1**
    - Causes:
        - Hypoventilation – **retains** CO_2 e.g. asthma after **exhaustion**, splinted diaphragm
        - Obstructive lung diseases e.g. chronic bronchitis (MCC), **CF**, late ARDS,
        - Upper airway obstruction – acute epiglottitis, croup
        - Respiratory muscle weakness – ALS, MG, GBS, poliomyelitis, phrenic N injury, hypokalaemia/hypophosphatemia (= less ATP).
        - Chest wall problems e.g. flail chest, ANK SPON, kyphoscoliosis,
        - CNS depression: narcotics (opioids), barbiturates, brainstem disease, trauma

- Metabolic acidosis
    - Bicarb **low** pH < 7.35 $\pm$ respiratory compensation (PaCo2 **low**)

A) Non-anion gap metabolic acidosis
- Aetiology based on anion gap. Anion gap = **(Na$^+$ + K$^+$) – (Cl$^-$ + HCO$_3^-$)**
- Important because any fall in bicarb will be compensated by increase in **Cl$^-$**
- 2 ways to **reduce** anion gap = reduce cations, or increase anions
    - Anions mainly albumin (high –ve charge), P, and S.
        - Therefore, hyperalbuminemia increases anion gap
    - **Multiple myeloma** = high IgG = cationic charge high $\rightarrow$ bind Na+ $\rightarrow$ low Na+ = increases anion gap
- If there is increased **unmeasured** anions e.g. Lac, ketoacids – then there is no increased in compensatory negative charges by Cl$^-$ and anion gap is **increased**.

B) Non-anion gap metabolic acidosis
- Causes:
    - Diarrhoea – MCC in children $\rightarrow$ loses bicarb in stool (pancreatic source and bile). *Cholestyramine resin* bind bicarb as well (and bile salts, drugs, and vitamin ADEK)
    - Acetazolamide – CA inhibitor $\rightarrow$ inhibit formation of bicarb (so reclamation and regeneration lost).
    - Spironolactone/ Addison's $\rightarrow$ loss of aldosterone effect (hypoaldosteronism) $\rightarrow$ H+ and K+ RETAINED (Na+ loss).
    - Saline infusion $\rightarrow$ volume expansion = RAAS inhibited = less aldosterone = less H+ secreted (reverse of contraction alkalosis). Hyperchloraemic metabolic acidosis
    - Hyperalimentation (e.g. TPN, IV nutrition) $\rightarrow$ metabolism of these nutrition creates HCl = reduce pH
    - Pancreatic fistula (chronic pancreatitis) – loss of bicarb rich fluid = hyprechloraemic metabolic acidosis.
    - Ammonium chloride ingestion – converted in liver to urea, consuming bicarb.
    - **RTA** – accumulation of acid in body as kidney cannot properly acidify urine

C) Anion gap metabolic acidosis
- Caused by increase in unmeasured anion. Causes = **MUDPILES CAT**
    - **M**ethanol – found in antifreeze, windshield wipers, solvents, moonshine. After metabolised by alcohol dehydrogenase – formic acid forms $\rightarrow$ visual loss and coma. Tx: fomepizole (inhibit alcohol dehydrogenase; in the past IV ethanol is used to compete).

- o Uraemia – urea and Cr accumulates e.g. <u>advanced</u> renal disease – where organic acids cannot be excreted at all. Hence P, S, urea all retained → anion gap. ***Aminoglycosides* contribute.**
  Urate as well (from renal failure)
- o **D**KA – in TIDM → triggered by infections, missed insulin dose, and other stresses (because insulin requirements of tissue cannot be met) → over-compensation by excess FA metabolism and ketone synthesis → ketoacids (acetoacetate + β-hyroxybutyrate). Tx: insulin + IVF + K^+ (insulin drives K^+ in).
- o **P**ropylene glycol → found in antifreeze as well; is converted into pyruvate, acetate, and lactate (acids). It contributes to seizures and coma when OD (CNS depression).
- o **I**ron tablets/ isoniazid
  - ▪ Fe poisoning → ferric iron ($Fe3+$) → CV toxicity → hypoperfusion and shock → lactic acidosis. Tx: supportive (ABCDE = O2 + IVF); lavage sometimes considered; if serious enough deferoxamine IV to chelate $Fe3+$
  - ▪ INH causes seizures → lactic acidosis.
- o **L**actic acidosis – lactate formed from pyruvate in many stress states e.g. sepsis, hypoxia/ischaemia, seizures, exercise, and also **METFORMIN treatment** in **renal failure.** Other causes are **theophylline OD, cyanide,** CO poisoning, & **congenital heart diseases**
- o **E**thylene glycol→ also found in antifreeze, solvents, and cleaners. Alcohol dehydrogenase metabolises it into **glycolate** and **oxalate** – both slowly excreted but are nephrotoxic. Oxalate precipitate to form **calcium oxalate renal stones.**
- o **S**alicylate – as discussed.

4. ENDOCRINOLOGY

GENERAL TIPS
- Endocrinology is a specialty of diagnostic tests – you should know how to interpret each of them.

- You should be able to differentiate the neck lumps!

- Diabetic medications, complications, and emergencies are essential points to commit to memory

THYROID ISSUES

Thyroid function tests: differentials
- Hypothyrodisim → high TSH, low T4
- Subclinical hypothyroidism (or Tx-ed hypothyroid) → high TSH, normal T4
- TSHoma → high TSH, high T4
- Hyperthyroidism → low TSH, high T4/3
- Sick euthyroid (or pituitary issue) → low TSH, low T4/3
- Normal TSH + abnormal T4 → ?artefact (TBG, amiodarone

Thyroid function tests: differentials
- Thyrotoxicosis → signs and symptoms of high sympathetic output (incld. diarrhoea)
  - **Tests:** TSH (then add T3/4); thyroid autoAb; isotope scan if cause unclear
  - Beta blocker for Sx
  - Anti-thyroid → "block" = carbimazole **1st choice** and PTU, and "replace" w levothyroxine; 131-Iodine; thyroidectomy
    - S/E carbimazole = rash, pruritus, over-Tx hypothyroid, **teratogenic** (fetal goitre), **agranulocytosis**
  - THYROID STORM (goitre, acute abdomen, heart failure = high output; precipitated by recent surgery = leak thy, recent Iodine ablation, anaestheisa, labour, contrast (contains Iodine), stresses)
    - IV fluids
    - Carbimazole (PO/NG) or Lugol's iodine
    - Hydrocort/dex (*prevents peripheral conversion T4 to T3)*
    - Digoxin/BB (propranolol) for arrhythmias (if asthmatic try esmolol = ultra-short acting or CCB = diltiazem)
    - Tx underlying cause e.g. infections

Grave's	DIFFUSE goitre Circulating IgG TSHR stimulating autoantibodies This can cross placenta to cause fetal thyrotoxicosis → must be treated e.g. PTU (cross placenta less) Associated with **autoimmune diseases** and additional signs from GAG deposition: • Eye disease = exophthalmos → less blinking = Stellwag sign (Tx: stop smoking, prism, high-dose steroids, decompression, orbital XRT) • Pretibial myxoedema above lateral malleoli • Thyroid acropachy (N.B. lid retraction, lid lag = Von Graefe sign are not specific to Graves).
Toxic multinodular goitre	NODULAR goitre Most common goitre in UK; can cause mass effect = compress e.g. retrosternal goitre Patients usually euthyroid but suddenly becomes thyrotoxic due to TSH-independent nodules developing Tx: surgery
Toxic adenoma	Solitary T3/4 producing nodule; "hot" on isotope scan
Subacute (de QUervain's) thyroiditis	Self-limiting PAINFUL goitre post-viral (tempts) Low (cold) isotope uptake on scan Tx = NSAIDs

Amiodarone can cause either hypo or hyperthyroidism (check TFTs every 6 months).

- Hypothyroidism→ signs and symptoms of LOW sympathetic output + coarse face
  - **Tests:** TSH (then add T3/4); thyroid autoAb.
  - Chol raised; macrocytic anaemia; signs of CCF (fluid overload)
  - Causes:
    - Primary – worldwide = deficiency; autoimmune e.g. **Hashimoto's** *(diffuse goitre due to TPO autoab; risk of conversion to marginal zone B-cell lymphoma);* **Riedel's fibrosing thyroidits** *(IgG4 disease -> hard as wood goitre fixed to neck, mimicking anaplastic carcinoma; signs of other IgG4 disease e.g. retroperitoneal fibrosis, liver disease. Tx = steroids ± surgery);* **post-Tx; drug-induced (Li+, amiodarone)**
    - Secondary – not enough TSH from hypopituitarism (uncommon)
  - MYXOEDEMATOUS COMA
    - Hypothermia, hyporeflexia. low BM, bradycardic, pancreatitis, psychosis/seizures → coma
    - PPt: recent radioiodine/thyroidectomy/pit surgery; infections; stresses
    - Tx: ventilate, replace (T3, glucose, warming); treat underlying cause (e.g. hypopit → steroids)

- OTHER neck lumps
  - Pharyngeal pouch → older man with dysphagia + halitosis + regurgitation → aspiration (posteromedial herniation)
  - Thyroglossal cyst → midline between thyroid isthmus and hyoid bone – move with tongue protrusion
  - Branchial cyst → TEENS with oval, mobile cyst between SCM and pharynx. Increase in size after URTI.
  - Cystic hygroma → baby < 2y w LEFT large transilluminating lump

- Thyroid cancer
  - Red flag = stridor, persistent cough, hoarseness, haemoptysis, lymphadenopathy, rapid growth, painless, fixed/hard lump
  - Step 1: measure TFT + clinical exam
  - Step 2: if step 1 suspicious (euthyroid or/and lymphadenopathy) → FNA (not ultrasound because you need a **histological Dx**)

Papillary CA (60% = MC)	**Younger** pt. Spread *locally* to **LN and lung** (jugulo-diagastric node met is the so-called lateral aberrant thyroid) Tx: **total thyroidectomy** to remove non-obvious tumour $\pm$ node excision $\pm$ ^{131}I to ablate residual cells. Give levothyroxine to suppress TSH. Prognosis: better if young and W.
Follicular ($\leq$ 25%)	Occurs in **middle-age** and spread early via **blood (bone, lungs)**!. Well-differentiated. Tx: **total thyroidectomy** + T_4 suppression + **radioiodine ablation**
Medullary (5%)	Sporadic (80%) vs. MEN2 syndromes ▢ perform phaeo screen pre-op; screen for *RE*. May produce **calcitonin** as tumour marker. Bx: calcitonin as localised amyloidosis in thyroid stroma. Don't concentrate iodine. Tx: total thyroidectomy + node clearance. External beam XRT may prevent regional recurrence.
Lymphoma (5%)	W: M = 3: 1. Pt: stridor or dysphagia. Do full staging pre-treatment = chemoXRT. Assess histology for MALT origin (associated w good prognosis) Tx: chemoXRT
Anaplsatic (Rare)	W: M = 3: 1. And elderly. Rapidly growing and hard invasive structure ▢ SOB, dysphagia, hoarseness. Poor response to ANY treatment. In absence of unresectable disease, excision + XRT to palliate (protect A).

PARATHYROID ISSUES

Hyperparathyroidism

- **Primary** (80% adenoma, >19% hyperplasia, <1% cancer)
  - ○ Pt: asymptomatic, with hypercalcaemic Sx (bones, stones, groans, psych overtones). Hypertension.
  - ○ Associations:
    - **MEN-1 (AD)** – *MEN1* tumour suppressor gene codes menin. **3 Ps**
      - Parathyroid adenoma/hyperplasia
      - Pituitary adenoma (acromegaly or prolactinoma)
      - Pancreas tumour (gastrinoma, insulinoma)
      - Others: carcinoid and adrenal tumours
    - **MEN-2A (AD)** – *ret* proto-oncogene mutation
      - Parathyroid hyperplasia (80%)
      - **Thyroid medullary CA (100%)** – prophylactic resection
      - Phaeochromocytoma (50%; bilateral)
    - Hyperparathyroid-jaw tumour syndrome (AD) – triad of disfiguring jaw fibromas, pituitary adenoma/cancer, and GU tumours.

MEN-2B – *ret* proto-oncogene
- ⬜ NO parathyroid hyperplasia
- ⬜ Thyroid – MTC
- ⬜ Adrenal – phaeo
- ⬜ Mucosal neuromas (= bumps on lips, cheeks, tongue, glottis, eyelids, and visible corneal nerves)
- ⬜ Marfanoid appearance

- **Secondary** (e.g. to vitamin D, CKD) → Tx: underlying cause, Phosphate binders, vitamin D replacement, *rarely: cinacalcet if high PTH and parathyroidectomy difficult.*

PRIMARY HYPERPTH	SECONDARY HYPERPTH
High Ca2+	Low/normal Ca2+
Low Pi	High Pi
High or inappropriately normal-high for that level of Ca2+	High PTH
High ALP	High ALP
Tx: Mild – fluids, avoid thiazides Mod – excise adenoma or all *hyperplastic* glands (if bone disease, high Ca2+, stones, reduced eGFR, age < 50). Complications: ○ HypoPTH – can save 1 gland ○ Hungry bone syndrome = rapid	Tx: underlying cause, Pi binders, Vit D, rarely: cinacalcet if PTH ≥ 85 and parathyroidectomy not possible

hypoCa due to bone remodelling after PTH is suddenly suppressed (check Ca for 2 weeks post-op) ○ RLN damage = hoarseness Cinacalcet = calcimimetic = allosterically activate CaSR to increase PTH sensitivity.	

- **Tertiary** – high Ca2+ and VERY high PTH. Due to autonomous parathyroid glands that has adapted after prolonged secondary hyperparathyroidism (e.g. chronic renal failure **after transplant**)

Hypoparathyroidism
- Primary – PTH secretion reduced from gland failure (e.g. autoimmune, surgical resection, hereditary)
  - ○ **Low Ca2+, high P, <u>ALP normal</u>, low PTH**
  - ○ **Pt:** hypocalcaemia = SPASMODIC = Spasms, Perioral paraesthesia, Anxiety/agitation, Seizures, Muscle tone high = colic, wheezing, dysphagia, Orientation impaired (confused), Dermatitis, Impetigo herptiformis (pustules in pregnancy), Chvostek's/Chorea/Cataracts/Cardiomyopathy/long QTc
    - ▪ **Trousseau sign of latent tetany** = carpopedal spasm on inflating BP cuff
    - ▪ **Chvostek sign** = facial muscle spasm on tapping CN VII near tragus
  - ○ **Associations:** APECED (autoimmune polyendocrinopathy e.g. Addison's/hypoPTH, candidiasis, ectodermal dysplasia), **DiGeorge syndrome** (CATCH-22: cardiac, abnormal facies, thymic hypoplasia, cleft palate, hypoCa2+, Chromosome 22)
  - ○ **Tx:** replace with alfacalcidol; may need Ca2+ gluconate infusion if very low
- Pseudohypoparathyroidism e.g. Albright's osteodystrophy
  - ○ GNAS1 mutation from mum (imprinting) in type 1A
  - ○ SHORT 4th and 5th fingers + round face + dental hypoplasia + short + low IQ
  - ○ **Low Ca2+, high P, high PTH** (normal-high ALP)

Familial hypocalciuric hypercalcaemia AR defect in CaSR (sensing receptor). Excess renal Ca2+ reabsorption → high serum Ca2+ Tests: Ca/Cr ratio < 1/100. Usually slightly elevated Ca2+ only = no Tx needed.

HYPOTHALAMUS-PITUITARY-ADRENAL AXIS ISSUES

Pituitary tumours
- Acidophil = GHoma, prolactinoma
- Basophil = ACTHoma
- Chromophobe = non-secretory
- In all – can cause pressure effect → headache, **bilateral temporal hemianopia** (superior field lost 1st from *inferior* compression c.f. craniopharyngioma), diabetes insipidus and effects to hypothalamic centres of temperature, sleep, appetite. Erosion to sella → CSF rhinorrhoea.
- Can give Sx via their hormones or lack of:
  - **Prolactinoma** most common

Hyperprolactinaemia and prolactinoma
- **Prolactin** = dopamine inhibiting factor
- **Causes:** physiological (pregnancy, stress, breastfeeding); drugs (MCC): dopamine antagonists (metoclop, haloperi, risperidone, etc.); oestrogen; diseases (prolactinoma, hypothalamic disease, trauma/surgery = stalk damage etc.)
- **Pt:**
  - Galactorrhoea + amenorrhoea in female
  - Male ASx – erectile dysfunction + less facial hair
  - Both late Cx: mass effect as above; osteoporosis
- **Dx:** always do a PREGNANCY test in females (DDx amenorrhoea), basal prolactin (confounded by stress, macroprolactinaemia = IgG-bound prolactin falsely +Ve ASx patients), *MRI* head
- **Tx of**
  - **Microprolactinoma < 1 cm** → DA antagonist e.g. bromcriptine (S/E: N, depression, postural hypotension – so give at night); carbegoline (more effective for Sx and fewer S/E but unsure if safe in pregnancy). **BOTH** are ergot alkaloids → so can rarely cause cardiac fibrosis (monitor with echo)
  - **Macroprolactinoma > 1 cm or visual field threatened** → surgery ± XRT

  - **ACTH – Cushing, GH – acromegaly** (see below), **FSH** – macro-orchidism (see Book 2).
  - **Hypopituitarism** (e.g. pituitary apoplexy = infarction; Sheehan syndrome – apoplexy from post-partum blood lost)
    - **Pt:** Addison's, hypos + SOB (GH loss), absent lactation, amenorrhoea + infertile + impotence, hypothyroid,; late: osteoporosis.
    - **Tx:** replace – hydrocort, thyroxine, somatotropin, testosterone or oestrogen or gonadotropin
    - **DDx:** Kallmann syndrome = anosmia + colour blindness + hypogonadotropic hypogonadism

Acromegaly
- F = M. 5% associated w MEN-1.
- Excess GH stimulates bone and soft tissue growth through increased IGF-1.

- **Symptoms**
  - Acroparaethesia
  - Amenorrhoea
  - Low libido
  - Headache
  - Increased sweating
  - Snoring (**OSA**)
  - Arthralgia + backache.
  - Curly hair
  - Weight gain
  - "My rings, shoes, hat done fit"
  - Wonky bite (malocclusion, prognathism)
  - "Used to be all muscle – now look haggard"

- Signs (often predates Dx by > 4y. If acromegaly occurs before bony epiphyses fuse = gigantism).
  - Large spade-like hands, jaw, and feet (sole may encroach dorsum)
  - Coarsened facies, wide nose
  - Big supraorbital ridges
  - Macroglossia (big tongue)
  - Widely spaced teeth
  - Thickened skin
  - Skin darkening
  - Acanthosis nigricans
  - Puffy lips, eyelids, and skin (oily and large-pored)
  - Skin tags
  - Widely spaced teeth
  - Scalp folds (*cutis verticis gyarta* – due to expanding but tethered skin)
  - Laryngeal dyspnoea (fixed cords)
  - OSA
  - Goitre (high thyroid vascularity)
  - Hepatomegaly
  - Proximal weakness + arthropathy
  - Carpal tunnel signs in 50%
  - Signs of pituitary mass (hypopituitarism, epilepsy, mass effect e.g. VA low, hemianopia)

- Cx (may pt w **CHF** or **DKA**)
  - Impaired glucose tolerance – 40%, DM in 15%.
  - Vascular – HTN, LVH ($\pm$ dilatation/CHF), cardiomyopathy, arrhythmias. There is increased risk of ischaemic heart disease and stroke (due to HTN $\pm$ insulin resistance and GH-induced increase in fibrinogen and decrease in protein S).
  - Neoplasia – **increased CRC risk** (colonoscopy may be needed).
- **Tests:**
  - BM
  - Ca^{2+} & PO_3^{4-} (parathyroid stimulation = high serum + urine calcium, high serum phosphate)
  - **IGF-1** gold standard blood test.
  - **OGTT** is still needed if baseline serum GH is > 0.4 mcg/L (1.2 mIU/L) and/or if high **IGF-1**
    - Normally GH secretion inhibited by high BM, and GH hardly detectable. In acromegaly, failed to suppress.
    - If lowest GH value during OGTT is above 1 mcg/L (3 mIU/L), acromegaly confirmed.
      - With general use of very sensitive assays, it has been said that this cut-off be decreased to 0.3 mcg/L (0.9 mIU/L).
  - GH (do not rely on random GH, as secretion pulsatile during peaks acromegalic, and normal levels overlap. GH also raised in stress, sleep, puberty, and pregnancy).
    - Collect samples for GH glucose at 0, 30, 60, 90, 120, 150 min.
    - Possible FP: puberty, pregnancy, hepatic, and renal disease, AN, and DM.
  - MRI scan of pituitary fossa
  - Look for hypopituitarism

- o VF and VA
- o ECG, echo
- o Old photos if possible.
- ☐ Tx:
  - o **1st line: transsphenoidal surgery:** aim to correct (or prevent) tumour compression by excising lesion, and to reduce GH and IGF-1 levels to at least "safe" level
  - o If surgery **fails** to correct GH/IGF-1 hypersecretion/**unfit**, try somatostatin analogues (SSA), and/or XRT, SSA being generally preferred.
    - ☐ Example: *octreotide* (Sandostatin LAR given q1m IM) or *lanreotide* (Somatuline LA). **S/E:** pain at injection site, GI, abdo cramps, flatulence, loose stools, GS, impaired glucose tolerance.
    - ☐ GH antagonist e.g. **pegvisomant** (rGH analogue = antagonist at the receptor) used if resistant or intolerant to SSA. It suppresses IGF-1 to normal in 90% **but** GH levels may rise... rarely tumour size increases – so monitor closely.
  - o XRT – if unsuitable to surgery or as an *adjuvant*. May **take years to work**.

Hyponatremia

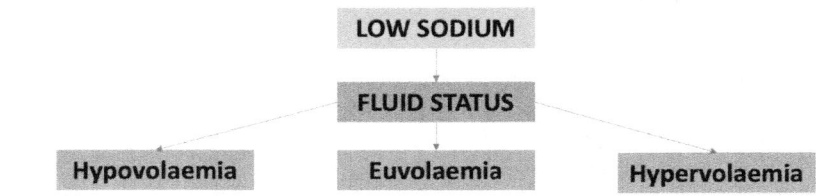

5 CAUSES

1. Diuretics
2. Inherited kidney disorders
3. GI loss (D/V)
4. Skin loss (burns or sweat)
5. Mineralocorticoid deficiencies

4 CAUSES

1. SIADH
2. Hypothyroidism
3. Short-term diuretics
4. SECONDARY adrenal insufficiency

3 CAUSES "Failures"

1. Heart failure
2. Renal failure (+ nephrotic)
3. Liver failure

SIADH

- Diagnosis is **of exclusion** where patient is **euvolaemic**; *inappropriately* high urine Na > 20, high urine Osm > 100 despite **hypoNa+ and low serum hypo-Osm**
- Because ADH excess = more *free* water reabsorbed by AQP2 → concentrated urine
- Causes: SMALL cell lung cancer & other cancers (prostate, lymphoma); chest (TB, PNA, mech ventilation); surgery; CNS (stroke, SAH, infections); drugs (SSRIs, psychotropics, opiates, nicotine, cytotoxics)
- Tx: **fluid restriction**; demeclocycline = tetracycline inhibit ADH production

Diabetes insipidus

- Polyuria + dipsia = dehydration
- Nephrogenic DI – impaired ADH response by kidney
  - **Causes**: LITHIUM, demeclocycline (SIADH Tx), CKD, low K+, high Ca2+, post-obstructive uropathy
- Cranial DI – reduced ADH secretion from *posterior pituitary gland*
  - **Causes**: Idiopathic (MCC), congenital (Wolfram's), brain tumour/bleed/ infection/ infiltration (sarcoidosis)
- DDx: psychogenic polydipsia
- Test to differentiate = BMs (DDx: DM); **water deprivation test (8h):**
  - Step 1 (Dx DI):
    - Normal = concentrated urine (Osm > 600)
    - PP = may be slightly less concentrated urine (400-600)
    - DI = diluted urine (Osm < 600)
  - Step 2: (NDI vs CDI):
    - Desmopressin IM and water can be drunk
    - Urine Osm for next 4 hours
      - CDI – kidneys respond = urine Osm > 600 (**treated**)
      - NDI – no increase (response) to ADH analogue
        - NDI Tx: thiazides, NSAID, underlying cause

Cushing's syndrome and disease
- Cushing syndrome = state of chronic glucocorticoid excess
- ACTH production will lead to **pigmentation** as alpha-melanocyte stimulating hormone is produced from its cleavage.
- Causes of Cushing <u>syndrome</u>
  - ACTH-dependent
    - Cushing disease = bilateral adrenal hyperplasia from **ACTH-secreting pituitary adenoma**
    - Ectopic ACTH production (small cell lung cancer, carcinoid) → pigmentation
    - Ectopic CRF production (very rare) – paraneoplastic as well
  - ACTH-independent
    - Iatrogenic **(MOST COMMON CAUSE)** – steroids
    - Adrenal adenoma – autonomous production so cortisol not suppressed by dex; abdo pain + female virilisation
    - Carney complex, McCune-Albright syndrome
- **Key presentation:**
  - Proximal weakness, recurrent Achilles tendon rupture, mood changes, acne, and sexual dysfunction (hirsutism, irregular menses, virilisation)
  - Lemon on a stick → truncal obesity with thin limbs; purple striae.
  - Buffalo hump (supraclavicular fat pad), moon facies, plethora
  - Osteoporosis, hypertension, insulin resistance
  - Signs of underlying disease = abdo mass, or visual field defect
- **Key findings: hypertension, LOW K+, metabolic alkalosis, high Na+** (opposite of ACE-inhibitors), *hyperglycaemia*
- **Key tests to differentiate causes of Cushing syndrome**
  - 1st line (screen): Overnight dexamethasone suppression test (outpatient) – failure to suppress cortisol; 24 hour urine cortisol – hard as outpatient (inpatient with catheter)
  - 2nd line:
    - 48 hour low-dose dex – confirmation of failure to suppress cortisol
    - 48 hour high-dose dex – DDx pituitary from other causes (pituitary causes will be suppressed)
  - CT adrenals, MRI pituitary

Diagnosis	ACTH levels	Low-dose dex	High-dose dex	Imaging/Tx
Cushing DISEASE (ACTH producing tumour)	High	Not suppressed	Suppression > 50%	Bilateral adrenal **hyperplasia** (CT); pituitary adenoma (MRI. **Tx:** transphenoidal <u>or</u> bilateral adrenalectomy if can't find source.
Ectopic ACTH	High	Not suppressed	Not suppressed	Bilateral adrenal **hyperplasia** (CT); **Tx:** find tumour, resect
Primary adrenal adenoma/CA	Low (ACTH-independent); high cortisol	Not suppressed (not necessary).	Not suppressed (not necessary).	Bilateral **ATROPHY** (CT) **Tx:** adrenalectomy
Exogenous steroids	Low (ACTH-independent); low cortisol	**Dx** is clinical. Tx: taper off steroids. Bilateral adrenal atrophy.		

- Tx:
    - Stop steroids if possible
    - Removal of pituitary gland by transsphenoidal surgery
    - Removal of adrenal glands (cures adenoma but not cancer; can also be used in refractory Cushing's disease despite pituitary removal; or if source unlocated)
        - **Nelson's syndrome:** bilateral adrenalectomy performed before treating pituitary tumour leads to disinhibition (lack of negative feedback) of that tumour → aggressive ACTH-secreting tumour growth → hyperpigmentation, VF defect/ophthalmoplegia, and *paradoxical worsening Cushing's*
    - Ectopic ACTH can be controlled by AZOLE drugs & mifepristone if tumour has not been located yet.

Addison's disease

- State of low glucocorticoid and mineralocorticoid (opposite of Cushing's and Conn's)
- Primary = destruction of cortex
    - 80% of causes in the UK is **autoimmune**
    - Secondary = TB (originally *described*); lymphoma; mets; infection; haemorrhage (**Waterhouse-Friderichsen syndrome**), congenital
- Secondary = iatrogenic (steroids withdrawal acutely)
- Presentation
    - Vague symptoms – constitutional
    - **Unexplained** N&V + abdo pain + diarrhoea/vomiting + dizziness/weakness
    - Vascular collapse and coma if acute (**Addisonian crisis**)
    - Tanned, pigmented palmar creases, buccal mucosa, and darkened scars (high ACTH = high α/γ–MSH)
    - Psych = depression, psychosis, anorexia
- **Key findings: HYPOtension, HIGH K+, metabolic acidosis, LOW Na+** (like ACE-inhibitors), *hypoglycaemia, AKI (poor urine output – pre-renal from hypotension)*
- **Key test:** short synACTHen stimulation test
    - Attempt to see if body can respond to synthetic ACTH
    - Plasma cortisol checked early in **early morning at 9 AM**, then 30 mins and 1 hour after. Expect cortisol to go up if able to produce cortisol... (False positive = steroids, COCP, pregnancy; stop steroids evening before).
    - If do not go up – suspect Addison's and find the cause: e.g. autoantibodies (21-hydroxylase adrenal antibodies)
    - If autoAb negative → CT adrenals etc.
- Tx:
    - ACUTE crisis → glucose, IVF, hydrocort +/- fludrocort
    - Non-acute → steroid replacement +/- mineralocort if postural hypotension

Conn's syndrome

- Primary hyperaldosteronism due to aldosterone producing adrenal adenoma (2/3 cases; 1/3 from bilateral hyperplasia)
- Triad of hypokalaemia, metabolic alkalosis, and hypertension
- Key labs: **LOW renin (Suppressed) and high aldosterone**
- Localisation: CT/MRI → if unilateral adenoma seen, *adrenal vein sampling*
- **Tx of Conn's = lap adrenalectomy** + spironolactone
- (Tx hyperplasia – medical w spironolactone or amiloride; Tx cancer – surgery)

Phaeochromocytoma

- Rule of 10s
  - 10% extra-adrenal, 10% malignant, 10% bilateral, 10% FHx
- FHx:
  - MEN2A
  - MEN2B
  - NF1 – schwannoma, plexiform neurofibroma, Lisch nodules, optic glioma, *café au lait (> 6) spots, axillary + inguinal freckling*
  - Von Hippel Lindau – phaeochromocytoma; haemangioblastoma of cerebellum, brainstem, spine; **RCC**; pancreatic cysts.
  - Sturge-Weber syndrome
- Classic triad of headache, sweating, tachycardia (sense of impending doom)
- Other presentation:
- Tests: 24 hours urinary **metanephrines**
- **Localisation:** abdominal CT/MRI, isotope scan
- **Tx:** surgery
  - **Pre-op blockade: strict alphabetical order** – alpha block then beta block to avoid crisis from unopposed alpha-adrenergic stimulation
  - **Emergency Tx:** alpha block with phentolamine (short-acting) then phenoxybenzamine (long-acting). Beta blocker added after this stage before surgery.

DIABETES AND GLUCOSE DISORDER

Type 1 DM	Type 2 DM
1st presented as symptomatic (younger) – sudden polyuria/dipsia, recurrent UTIs, thrush, and *weight loss*.	Usually asymptomatic – incidental. Weight *gain* (obese), gradual onset.
Insulin-dependent autoimmune disease (GADA, ICA, HLADR3/4). **Therefore, low C-peptide**.	Non-insulin dependent due to end-organ insulin resistance (eventual deficiency) – **therefore, initially normal C-peptide**
DKA	HHS

- Diagnostic criteria (WHO)
    - ○ **Asymptomatic patients must have TWO abnormal readings**
    - ○ **Symptomatic patients may only need ONE**
    - ○ HbA1C > **6.4%** (47 mmol/l)
        - Should be repeated every 3 months – turnover glycated Hb
        - To convert % to digit: % **minus** 2 for first digit; % **minus** 4 for 2nd digit e.g. 9% = 75 mmol/l (9-2; 9-4).
        - **Cannot use in** Type 1 DM (as on insulin = body will respond well = falsely low end-glycation products), young kids (use a **random** glucose instead), less than 2 months symptoms **(turnover RBC 3 months)**, iron deficient anaemia, haemolytic anaemia or haemoglobinopathies or malaria, HIV (due to ART treatment affecting RBC lifespan), pregnancy (or pregnant in past 2 months), pancreatic damage, *liver/renal failure* (rapid RBC turnover).
    - ○ OGTT 2 hours > **11.1**
    - ○ Fasting glucose > **7.0**
    - ○ Random glucose > **11.1**
- Definitions
    - ○ Impaired glucose tolerance: **7.8 – 11.1** and normal fasting glucose
    - ○ Impaired fasting glucose: **5.5 – 7** and normal OGTT
- Diagnostic uncertainty:
    - ○ GADA, beta-islet cells antibodies, *low* C-peptide, *high* ketones → type 1

Special diabetes
- Latent autoimmune diabetes in adult (**LADA**) – type 1 DM i.e. autoimmune but present later as an adult instead of younger age. C-peptide undetectable.
- Maturity onset of diabetes of young (**MODY**) – autosomal dominant type 2 DM presents younger rather than older (<25y). C-peptide detectable over years. Usually do not require insulin but may have urogenital tract malformations.
- **Wolfram syndrome (DIDMOAD)** = Diabetes Mellitus + Optic Atrophy < **16 years old**. Associated with Dabetes Insipidus, sensorineural Deafness, urogenital tract malformations, and neurology (ataxia, seizures, neuropathies).
- Other causes: drugs (STEROIDS, ART for HIV, Thiazides, anti-psychotics), infection (CMV, rubella), pancreatic (inflammation, trauma, surgery, CF, or haemochromatosis = bronze diabetes), endocrine (Cushing's, acromegaly, phaeochromocytoma, hyperthyroidism, glucagonoma, pregnancy)

Diabetic ketoacidosis vs Hyperosmolar hyperglycaemic state

DKA	HHS
Type 1 DM	Type 2 DM
Despite high glucose, the lack of insulin prevents its utilisation. Therefore, body pushed to starvation state, forcing ketoacidosis to produce energy	There is *some* insulin in type 2 diabetics so no ketone metabolism switch. Main issue is dehydration + hyperglycaemia → hyperosmolality. <ul><li>**Early shift** – ECF hyperosmolar (water shift ICF→ ECF)</li><li>**Late phase** – continued osmotic diuresis (volume loss = dehydration = hyperosmolality)</li><li>* Insulin Tx without adequate IVF → shift glucose from ECF to ICF = hypotension and cerebral oedema</li></ul>
More acute (days)	More insidious (weeks)
Vomiting, drowsiness, dehydration with polyuria/dipsia/fatigue; Kussmaul respiration (hyperventilation to blow out CO_2 due to metabolic acidosis) and fruity breath (ketones)	Precipitant (infection, cardiovascular) → polyuria/polydipsia over weeks = dehydrated... **Mainly neurological signs (FND, VA changes, confusion, coma)**. No fruity breath.
Acidaemia pH < 7.3/bicarb < 15 Hyperglycaemia BM > 11 (or known DM) Ketonemia $\geq$ 3 or ketonuria ++	Hypovolaemia Marked hyperglycaemia > 30 **&** no ketonaemia < 3 **or** acidosis pH >7.3, bicarb > 15 Osm > 320 usually
Fixed rate insulin (50 soluble insulin to 50 ml saline at 0.1 unit/kg/h) to replace insulin deficiency (continue basal insulin) But avoid hypos (**start dextrose 10% if gluc < 14**)	**Firstly, give IV FLUIDS (normal saline** – *ever. if high Na+*) with *no* **insulin over 48 hours** (up to 8-15L deficit) Replace K+ when peeing (K+ shift less pronounced because less acidosis/no ketones) *Only start insulin if BM falling 5 per hour with the rehydration (keep at least 10-15 in 1ˢᵗ 24 h to prevent cerebral oedema and vascular collapse)* *

Cx: cerebral oedema, aspiration pneumonia, VTE |(dehydration), hypoK+/Mg2+/P. HHS worse.
REFERENCE: www.abcd.care

Hypos (BM < 4)
- Autonomic Sx = sweating, anxiety/agitation, tremor, palpitations, dizziness, hunger
- Neuroglycopenic Sx = drowsy/confusion, visual issues, seizures, coma
- Tx
  - Conscious = sugary drink/sweets
  - Conscious + uncooperative/vomit = glucose gel (Hypostop) buccal
  - Unconscious or refractory to above → dextrose 10% → 20% → glucagon
  - Long-acting carb once BM >4 and patient recovered
  - Glucagon usage training with relatives to use in community
  - Do not omit basal insulin

- DVLA advice for hypos: stop car safely, switch engine off, eat fast-acting carbohydrate, wait 45 minutes before starting. To prevent – snack regularly if long journey. Do not delay meals.

Chronic complications of diabetes
- Injection site: lipohypertrophy, infections. Rotate sites.
- Other Cx are due to microvascular osmotic damage from high sugar levels
- Cardiovascular – atherosclerosis → higher MI risk (can be silent). *Diabetes have lower target BP especially if end-organ damage* (T1DM < 135/85; T2DM < 140/80; in **both** aim <130/80 if end-organ damage = microalbuminuria, retinopathy, etc.). **ACE-inhibitors preferred** except Afro-Caribbean as per NICE guidelines. **Aspirin used as secondary prevention (not primary prevention).**
- Renal – nephropathy (hyaline arteriosclerosis of efferent arterioles) – **microalbuminuria is first and most important sign. This reflects cardiovascular risk.** Dipstick CANNOT assess this – urine alb:Cr should be sent (>3 is positive). **ACE-inhibitors should be started** even if BP normal to prevent progression.
- Diabetic retinopathy; cataracts – *see Ophthalmology in Book 2*
- Diabetic neuropathies
  - Amyotrophy = proximal motor neuropathy = very painful progressive weakness with wasting (quads, butt). **Unilateral** usually. Absent knee DTRs.
  - Symmetrical sensory distal polyneuropathy = gloves and stocking distribution of paraesthesia. **Assessed with 10G monofilament fibre + vibration sense.**
  - Focal neuropathy = one nerve affected only e.g. CN VII
  - Mononeuritis multiplex = acute mononeuropathy (SENSORY AND MOTOR loss) of non-contiguous nerves → asymmetrical pattern.
  - **Autonomic neuropathy** → postural Sx, gustatory sweating, <u>impotence</u>, visual blurring, gastroparesis = full all the time (Tx: **metoclopramide prokinetic**)
  - **Neuropathic pain:** amitriptyline, gabapentin/pregabalin, or duloxetine ON
- Foot ulcers – due to combination of neuropathy, ischaemia, bony deformity (Charcot joint), and infections.
  - PVD – Doppler to check foot pulses. May need angioplasty/ stents/ amputations
  - Charcot joint – bed rest + orthotics (Cast/crutches) to settle oedema ± bisphosphonates
  - Cellulitis – admit for swab, blood cultures, XR (rule out osteomyelitis, IV antibiotics. 1st line = flucloxacillin (MC bug is staph).
- Dermatology:
  - Lipidoca diabeticorum – shiny, yellowish area on shin with vessels growth
  - Acanthosis nigricans
  - Granuloma annulare

Diabetic medications
- Aim HbA1C of 48 = 6.5%. Used in conjunction with lifestyle modification.
- Type I DM – insulin
- Type 2 DM: METFORMIN standard release 1st line
- If GI upset → metformin modified release 2nd line
- If still fail or HbA1C > 58 = 7.5%, consider first intensification

- o Metformin + sitagliptin
- o Metformin + pioglitazone
- o Metformin + sulphonylurea e.g. gliclazide
- o Metformin + dapagliflozin
- Second intensification if still fail (7.5%) – triple therapy (aiming at HbA1C 7% = 53).
- If need > 3 drugs – start insulin...

Type 2 diabetes – drugs summary:

Metformin	Insulin sensitisation – so only effective if residual islet cells left... Improve HbA1C 1-2% (same as lifestyle) with good M&M benefits. Stop weight gain. **No** hypos and dirt cheap. Therefore drug of 1st choice. S/E: **GI upset most common** (can try *modified release*), lactic acidosis (is mythical but deeply entrenched in teachings – so still stopped 2-3 days before surgery or contrast; risk factors: **dehydration**). For this reason, **eGFR < 30/Cr> 150, metformin is held/stopped.**
Glicazide (2nd gen)	K_{ATP} channel inhibitor = increase insulin secretion Improve HbA1C 1-2%. Causes <u>weight gain</u>, **hypos** (less so for 2nd generation) = **job implications.** 2nd line drug (if metformin contraindicated) or add-on Other S/E: rarely hepatic cholestasis, blood dyscrasias, and skin allergic reaction. Omitted in the morning of surgery.
Gliptins	DPP-4 inhibitor (increase GLP-1 endogenously) = insulin secretion *Slight* HbA1C reduction <1% Weight-neutral **No** hypo risk on its own (because it has a post-prandial effect by relying on endogenous GLP-1, which only release insulin when glucose present) Good 2nd line if eGFR > 50. Other S/E: mainly headaches > N&V, **heart failure, pancreatitis/ pancreatic CA risk**, infection risk, arthralgia.
Glitazones	PPAR-gamma activator = insulin secretion + increase sensitivity *Slight* HbA1C improvement < 1.5%. Weight **gain.** Use if insulin RESISTANT; better lipid profile and MI risk reduction. Also used if **NAFLD.** S/E and hence C/I are: **fluid retention = CCF**, *hepatotoxic*, **osteoporosis + fractures**, *bladder cancer*, drug interactions (sulpha allergy, metabolised by CYP450). Monitoring: LFTs every 2 months for 1 year. Monitor and stop in 3-6m if ineffective.
Gliflozins	Selective SGLT2 inhibitor = blocks glucose reabsorption by kidney = excess glycosuria... therefore only effective if eGFR > 60 Reduced mortality in patients with **cardiovascular disease and heart failure**. Weight **LOSS.** S/E: **NORMOGLYCAEMIC DKA, UTIs + thrush + diuresis (glycosuria)**, hyperkalaemia

Exenatide, liraglutide	Glucagon-like peptides (GLP) analogues/mimetics = augment insulin release and slow gastric emptying. Longer half-lives than endogenous incretins. **No hypos when used alone.** **WEIGHT LOSS** (less than insulin) – patient feels fuller from slow gatric emptying. HbA1C reduction <1%. **Doesn't improve CV outcomes.** Given 5 minutes S/C before meal. **Strict indications**: BMI > 35 + psych/medical problems associated w obesity <u>or</u> BMI < 35 for which insulin poses occupational implications or weight loss may benefit obesity comorbidities. **S/E:** THREE injections (TDS), mainly GI side effects *including pancreatitis/ pancreatic cancer risk* (similar to DPP4i), worsens diabetic gastroparesis (C/I). C/I in eGFR <30.
Repaglinide, nateglinide	Secretogogues = sulphonylurea receptor binders = increase insulin release HbA1C <1.5% reduction Rapid in onset and short duration of activity (given 30 mins before meal)... may be used in someone who has irregular meal times and poor BM control. Rash, N&V + GI upset, **hypos,** *hepatotoxic* (C/I). Rather disfavoured drug: "**Not loved, not NICEd, not livered**"
Acarbose	Intestinal alpha-glucosidase inhibitor = less starch breakdown = less absorption. Very small HbA1C benefit. Weight-neutral. Rarely used in **Type 1s** to reduce post-prandial hyperglycaemia and in **DUMPING SYNDROME**. S/E: **flatulence + abdo** discomfort + osmotic diarrhoea logically follows...
Orlistat	Inhibit pancreatic and gastric lipases = less fatty acid → steatorrhea and weight lost. NICE guidelines: BMI >28 + risk factors **or** BMI > 30. Should only continue > 3months if ≥ 5% weight lost evident.

- **Insulin**
  - Benefits: decrease HbA1C by 1.5 to 3.5% with **no dose limit;** titratable; rapid; improve lipid profile
  - Types
    - Ultra-fast acting (Novorapid = insulin aspart, Humalog)
    - Short-acting soluble insulin (Actapid, Humulin S)
    - Intermediate-acting (Humulin I, Insulatard)
    - Long-acting (**Lantus** = insulin glargine, *Levemir = insulin determir*)
    - Tuojeo = very concentrated insulin
    - Degludec = very long-acting (used OD for convenience)
    - **Pre-mixed insulins:**
      - NovoMix
  - Regimens
    - Biphasic → BD pre-mixed insulin.
      - Good for type 2 DM or regular lifestyle type 1 DM
    - Basal-bolus → QDS insulin (**long-acting morning, ultra-fast acting before each of 3 main meals)**
      - Good for type 1 DM to achieve flexible lifestyle

- o Physiological rise in BM = Dawn phenomenon – *physiologically* high BM early mornings (2-8AM), no nocturnal hypos due to falling insulin + rising cortisol/GH.
- o Scenarios in titration in **BD pre-mixed** insulin
    - ▪ If BM high lunchtime and teatime – 10% increase breakfast dose
    - ▪ If BM elevated before bed and before breakfast – 10% increase teatime/lunch dose.
- o Scenarios in titration in **basal-bolus** insulin
    - ▪ BM high lunchtime → increase breakfast dose 10%
    - ▪ BM high teatime → increase lunchtime dose 10%
    - ▪ BM high dinner time → increase evening meal dose
    - ▪ BM high breakfast → increase **basal** dose
- o Titration usually 10-20% of dose (usually 2-4 units steps)
- o Somogyi effect – high *rebound* BM in the morning due to **insufficient night-time** insulin delivery in **T1DM** → hypoglycaemia at night with compensatory surge of glucagon, cortisol, GH, adrenaline. **Tx: increase night-time dose.**
- o Sick day rules:
    - ▪ Check BM **QDS** and look for ketonuria
    - ▪ Increase insulin dose if BM rising (Stress hyper)
    - ▪ GP may consider ultra-fast acting insulin 6-8 unit
    - ▪ Admit if vomiting, dehydrated, ketotic-prone, children, or pregrant
- Driving advice: NOTIFY if on insulin or sulphonylureas **AND** >1 hypo in last 12 months, self-monitoring, not regularly reviewed. Stricter for **HGV drivers** (no hypos last 12m, full awareness of hypos, self-monitoring regularly – at least BD and times of driving)

Bariatric surgery and islet cell transplant
- *Bariatric surgery indications*: BMI $\geq$ 35 + 1 x comorbidity than can respond to weight loss; BMI 30 – 34.9 and recent-onset Type 2; xonsider for Asian origin with recent Type 2 onset at lower BMI than 30.
- **Dumping syndrome** post-fundoplication → bypass of food too rapidly = pancrease excrete too much insulin (early <30mins or late < 3h) → flushing, dizziness, shakiness (**hypos**) post-meal.
- *Islet cell TXP indications*: **type 1** DM $\geq$ 2 severe hypos in 2 years **and** impaired hypos. C/I = obese, uses >50U insulin/d, and poor renal function

Other glucose disorders
- Glucagonoma = flushes + diarrhoea (Differential = carcinoid), **diabetes**, DVT, depression, NME rash, **hyperglycaemia**, weight loss.
- Hypoglycaemic hyperinsulinaemia
    - o Insulinoma = high insulin (proinsulin) and C-peptide. **Associated with VHL and MEN 1.**
    - o Factitious disease/exogenous insulin poisoning – high insulin + low C-peptide (low pro-insulin)
    - o Factitious disease/Sulphonylureas overdose = high insulin + high C-peptide (= from endogenous insulin/pro-insulin cleavage). E.g. misuse in weightlifters for stamina). Drug levels mainly to DDx insulinoma.

5. GASTROENTEROLOGY AND HEPATOLOGY

> ## GENERAL TIPS
> - Nutritional deficiencies/diets, IBS, colitis, coeliac disease are often tested
>
> - Know the red flags for oesophageal/gastric cancers
>
> - You should be able to interpret liver function tests and hepatitis serology

OESOPHAGEAL ISSUES

Achalasia
- Degeneration of Auerbach's plexus – causing discoordinated peristalsis and lower sphincter failure of relaxation.
- Dysphagia for both solids and liquids → so halitosis & increased risk of SCC
- High pressure on manometry; Bird's beak (dilared tapering) of oesophagus on barium swallow
- Tx: CCB/nitrates; endoscopic dilation; Heller's myotomy

Anti-emetics in a nutshell
- Cyclizine (H1 antagonist) – emetogenic for GI (Post-op N/V = PONV) and vestibular causes
- Metoclopramide, haloperidol, domperidone, prochloperazine (D2 antagonist) – emetogenic for GI, vestibular, and **opiates** → S/Es: prokinetic (**not used in bowel obstruction**) & can cause **dystonias and oculogyric crises**.
- Ondansetron (5-HT3 antagonist) – emetogenic for chemotherapy and surgery
- Others: dexamethasone – adjunct e.g. induction of anaesthesia (reduces PONV) and brain mets

Acute upper GI bleed
- Rockall score – risk stratification (mortality). Done pre- and post-endoscopy.

Pre-endoscopy	0 pt	1 pt	2 pts	3 pts
Age	< 60 y	60 – 79 y	≥ 80 y	
Shock: SBP and HR	BP > 100 mmHg HR < 100 bpm	BP > 100 mmHg HR > 100 bpm	BP < 100 mmHg	
Co-morbidity	NIL major	Heart failure Ischaemic HD	Renal failure Liver failure	MET
Post-endoscopy Dx	*MW tear; no lesion; no signs of recent bleed*	*All other Dx*	*Upper GI malignancy*	
Signs of recent haemorrhage on endoscopy	*None, or dark red spot*		*Blood in upper GI tract; adherent clot; visible vessel (Dieulafoy lesion)**	

*Dieulafoy lesion = high-risk of bleed therefore change stratification to high risk

- Causes:

Mallory-Weiss syndrome	Persistent vomiting or retching causing mucosal tear → arterial bleed. *Self-limiting.* Complication = Boerrhaave syndrome – oesophageal rupture due to vomiting against closed glottis → think when shock + surgical emphysema (Hamman sign = crunching sound on auscultation due to mediastinal emphysema).
Peptic (gastric and duodenal ulcers)	**Gastric ulcer (pain with meals)** – *H. pylori,* smoking, NSAIDs/steroids, refluxed duodenal contents, delayed gastric emptying, burns (Curling's ulcer), neurosurgery (Cushing's ulcer) **Duodenal ulcer (pain after meals)** – **4X commoner.** *H.pylori,* smoking, NSAIDs/steroids, increased gastric emptying, blood group **O** Zollinger-Ellison syndrome – gastrin secreting adenoma. **Suspect when:** multiple ulcers of stomach and duodenum + FHx. Associated with **MEN 1** (= parathyroid adenoma = hypercalcemia = bones, stones, moans, psych overtones). **Measure gastrin levels,** scintigraphy (OctreoScan) if small to localise tumour. 20% have hepatic mets. Posterior duodenal ulcers – high risk as nearest to gastroduodenal artery and can erode into it. See management below (next section).
Varices	Secondary to portal hypertension; compounded by liver failing to synthesis vitamin K dependent clotting factors. Causes: • Pre-hepatic (thrombosis portal or splenic vein) • Intra-hepatic – cirrhosis, fibrosis, sarcoid, myeloproliferative disease • Post-hepatic – Budd Chiari hepatic vein thrombosis, right heart failure, constrictive pericarditis

- Other characteristics: urea out of proportion to Cr, melena
- Management
  - Airway, NBM
  - IVF + blood transfusion + correct clotting (e.g. FFP, PTCC; vitamin K; discontinue NSAIDs etc.)
  - **For suspected varices** – use terlipressin (vasoconstrict to reduce portal blood pressure; renoprotective… but vasoconstricts coronary vessels too → arrhythmias)
  - Abx cover
  - Once stable: urgent endoscopy within 12 hours for Dx and control of bleeding:

- Endotherapy – adrenaline, clips, or cauterisation (2 of 3); if varices – band ligation or sclerotherapy.
- If fail – embolization (IR) or surgery
- Sengstaken-Blakemore tube can tamponade varices after intubation
- For **varices**: trans-jugular intrahepatic portal systemic stenting (TIPS) – salvage therapy for refractory bleed after endoscopic failure.
  - If unstable: urgent surgery
  - **72 hours high dose IV infusion of PPI (Omeprazole)** as per Hong Kong protocol
  - Tx *H. pylori* (see below).

Omeprazole	1. Hyponatraemia, hypomagnesemia
	2. Diarrhoea (increased risk of *C. difficle* esp. if on Abx)
	3. Tubular interstitial nephritis (TIN)
	4. Osteoporosis in long-term
	5. Interacts with clopidogrel

GORD and dyspepsia
- GORD – heartburn after meals; water-brashing (salivation); **nocturnal asthma**; chronic cough and sore throat; sinusitis.
  - **Hiatus hernia** – mainly <u>sliding</u>; less common rolling (para-oesophageal; higher strangulation risk).
  - Lifestyle advice – stop smoking; small regular meals; reduce hot drinks/EtOH/ citrus/spicy foot/caffeine etc; avoid eating < 3h before bed; raise bed head
  - Drugs: antacids, PPI (best) → if refractory: add H2RA.
  - Surgery: Nissen fundoplication; hiatal hernia repair.

Ranitidine*,	1. Diarrhoea, GI upset
cimetidine,	2. Liver dysfunction
famotidfine (H2	3. **Cimetidine** inhibits liver CYP450... but not famotidine or
receptor antagonist)	ranitidine

*Removed from UK market due to contamination in 2019

- Dyspepsia
  - Causes: ulcers, GORD, oesophagitis/gastritis/ duodenitis, malignancy:
    - ALARM Sx (red flags; box) – 2WW, ?gastric CA
- Dx/Tx algorithm:
  - If ≥ 55y **and** persistent Sx <u>or</u> ALARMS => 2WW gastroscopy
  - If < 55y **and** no red flags
    - Treat as isolated dyspepsia first with LIFESTYLE changes + stop offending drug if able. **Review in 4 weeks.**
    - If no improvement → Test and Treat *H. pylori*
      - [13]C breath test **most accurate and non-invasive**

> Anaemia
> Loss of weight
> Anorexia
> Recent onset/progressive Sx
> Melaena/haematemesis
> Swallowing difficulties

- - **Triple therapy:** PPI + amoxicillin + clarithromycin/metⁿo **4 weeks**.
    - If still no improvement → check ^{13}C breath test again to confirm eradication. *If eradicated* – PPI or H_2RA for **4 weeks**. Consider OGD.
      - If not eradicated – try another triple therpay combination
    - If on PPI/H_2RA without improvement <u>and</u> eradicated **(total of 8-12 weeks)** → Consider OGD
- Tx for **ulcers** are similar: lifestyle, *H. pylori* eradication, stop offending drugs, PPIs +/- H2RA to allow ulcer healing. If haemorrhage or perforated (signs and symptoms of peritonitis) → surgery.
- *Functional* dyspepsia is common – PPIs, CBT, and low-dose amitriptyline ON may help.
- Dose of PPI may be increased in cases like Zollinger-Ellison syndrome or corrosive substance consumption.
  - In ZES, somatostatin analogues (Octreotide) and chemotherapy may be used.

Barrett's

- Metaplasia of stratified squamous **to** columnar epithelium from chronic acid irritation (GORD).
- Can transform to **adenocarcinoma** (risk of progression *low*).
- If no dysplasia and short < 3cm – discharge.
- High-grade dysplasia or carcinoma in situ → endoscopic resection or RF ablation
- Low-grade dysplasia → repeat endoscopy 6 months before Tx with RFA>
- Surveillance every 2-3 years if extensive disease ($\geq$ 3 cm).

COLITIS
Inflammatory bowel disease
- UC vs Crohn's

ULCERATIVE COLITIS	CROHN'S
Mucosal, submucosal (superficial)	Full-thickness w fissures (knife-like) and fistula
Rectum to caecum (continuous)	Mouth to anus (skip lesions)
LLQ pain w bloody diarrhoea (showy)	RLQ pain w non-bloody diarrhoea
Crypt abscesses w Nø	Lymphoid aggregates w granulomas
PSEUDO-polups; haustral loss (lead piping)	Cobblestoning, creeping fat, strictures (string-sing)
Smoking PROTECTS M (middle-aged)	Smoking increases risk M=F
Arthritis (ank spon etc.), uveitis, erythema NODOSUM, pyoderma gangrenosum. **PSC and p-ANCA**	Arthritis (ank spon etc.), uveitis, erythema NODOSUM, pyoderma gangrenosum. **Oxalate stones**
Toxic megacolon and CA	Malabsorption, fistula, CA

- Ulcerative colitis
  - **Truelove-Witts criteria** (modified)

Parameter	Mild UC	Moderate	Severe
Motions/day	≤ 4	5	≥ 6
PR bleed	Small	Moderate	Large
T°C	Apyrexial	$37.1 - 37.8\ ^{\circ}C$	$> 37.8\ ^{\circ}C$
Resting HR	< 70 bpm	70 – 90 bpm	> 90 bpm
Hb	> 110 g/L	105 – 110 g/L	< 105 g/L
ESR (do CRP too)	< 30		> 40 (or CRP > 45 mg/L)

  - UC maintenance:
    - Mild → 5-ASA (aminosalicyclates) e.g. **mesalazine** PR (if distal), PO more effective than steroids
    - Moderate → steroids to induce remission then maintain on 5-ASA. Monoclonal biologics (infliximab, adalimumab).
  - Severe/acute UC → admit, NBM, IVF, IV/PR steroids
    - Poor responders day 5 → ciclosporin or infliximab to avoid surgery
    - If fail to improve still → colectomy day 7
    - If fulminant colitis => toxic megacolon → urgent colectomy
  - UC surgery potentially curable in controlled disease

- Crohn's
  - Crohn maintenance (mild-moderate): steroids PO/PR (5-ASA does not work!); azathioprine/6-mercaptopurine > methotrexate. Biologics.
    - Immunomodulation used if cannot taper off steroid without flaring or if $\geq$ 2 flares/year
    - For azathioprine or 6-mercaptopurine – **assess thiopurine methytransferase/TPMT activity** before starting (do not offer if low or absent – use *MTX instead*)
    - Offer biologics if refractory (vedolizumab, ustekinumab, infliximab) – continue until treatment failure or surgery.
  - *Crohn flare or severe disease:* **IV steroids, IV fluids.** Do not offer 5-ASA.
  - Crohn's diet = LOFFLEX diet (low fat, fibre-limited exclusion)
  - > 50% need at least **1 surgery but in CD it NEVER cures** (CD affects gut to anus). The aims of surgery in CD are:
    - Resect affect areas without causing short bowel syndrome
    - Control perianal disease or fistula
    - Defunctioning (e.g. temporary ileostomy) to relive obstruction
- *Surveillance in IBD – colonoscopy.* **Offered to IBD colitis** Sx $\geq$ **10 years** (risk of CRC)
  - High risk: extensive active/severe disease (on histology/endoscopy), **PSC**, strictures, dysplasia, FHx < 50y of CRC → every 1y
  - Intermediate risk → extensive but mild active inflammation (histology/endoscopy), post-inflammatory polyps, FHx > 50y of CRC → every 3 years
  - Low risk: extensive but quiescent disease (or left-sided UC/Crohn's) → every 5 years

Infectious colitis

- *Clostridium difficile*
  - Profuse watery diarrhoea with characteristic smell → CDT (toxins) in stools.
  - **Raised CRP + WCC (marked neutrophilia up to 40) + low albumin**; pseudomembrane on endoscopy (adherent plaques on background of inflamed/oedematous non-ulcerated mucosa)
  - **Complication**: ileus → toxic megacolon (>5.5 cm) → perforation, MSOF (AKI, etc.)
  - **Drugs to avoid**: antibiotics (CIPROFLOXACIN > macrolides), PPIs (abolish acid defence to kill bacteria), anti-spasmodics
  - **Severe if**: WCC++++, use of anti-spasmodic, shock, previous infection, >70y
  - Tx: STOP offending drug
    - Mild-moderate: **metronidazole oral**
    - Severe (WCC > 15, AKI, colitis, T > 38.5°C_ : vancomycin ORAL + metronidazole IV
      - May need colectomy if not controlled
    - Recurrent or refractory disease: *findaxomicin* may be trialled.
  - PPx: **wash hands** with soap (EtOH gel do not kill spores), gloves, cleaning

Other causes of GI infection:
- Gastroenteritis → pre-formed toxin = rapid-onset 4-6 hours, VOMIT predominante; whereas *in vivo* toxin takes longer (incubation time). Invasion causes dysentery (blood diarrhoea).
- *Food poisoning is notifiable!* Food sources:
  - Campy → poultry
  - *Salmonella* → poultry and their uncooked eggs (e.g. mayo)
  - *S. aureus* → cream-based puddings or pastries; sliced deli meat/sandwiches
  - *B. cereus* → reheated rice/soup
  - *Listeria* → soft cheese from unpasteurised milk, refrigerated meat & pâté (& ready-to-cook meats, hot dogs), raw veg. **Advice to pregnany ladies!**
  - *E. coli* → soft cheese from unpasteurised milk, raw fruit and veg (Romaine lettuce incident), **undercooked ground beef** (beef burgers – should be cooked until juices run clear)
  - *Norovirus* → shellfish, infected food worker (touching ice, sandwiches etc.)

- Summary of key characteristics:

Norovirus	1 day incubation → acute D&V lasting 2+ days; very infectious – spread by contact, food (epidemics e.g. on cruise ships); notifiable. Dx: stool antigen
Rotavirus	1-3 day incubation →watery diarrhoea + vomiting for up to 1 week (longer period than norovirus). Dx: stool antigen. Live vaccine in childhood (2 doses aged 12 weeks and 8y).
Campylobacter jejuni	Incubation 2-5 days → dysentery + pain + headache Complications: sepsis, hepatitis, pancreatitis, miscarriage, **reactive arthritis, Gullian-Barre** ascending paralysis Tx: clarithromycin or ciprofloxacin
Salmonella	Non-typhoidal – incubation 6h to 3 days → dysentery + cramps. Complications: sepsis, meningitis, **osteomyelitis + septic arthritis** (sickle cell) Tx: ciprofloxacin or clarithromycin
Staph aureus	Pre-formed toxins → **30 minutes to 6 hours** → sudden V&D, cramps
Bacillus cereus	Spores reactivated by heat → **8h to 16 hours** → V&D. Self-limiting.
Listeria monocytogenes	Variable incubation (up to months) Vague flu-like symptoms → diarrhoea in more immunocompromised. Complications: abscess, endocarditis, **meningoencephalitis (extremes of age)**, pregnancy loss or preterm delivery (placentitis/aminoitis). **Tx: AMOXICILLIN**
E. coli	**O157:H7** → **Shiga-toxin** producing *E. coli* (STEC) → haemorrhagic colitis (dysentery). Complications: 10% **haemolytic uraemic syndrome** (verotoxin damages endothelial cells and causes thrombin deposit → microangiopathy haemolytic anaemia picture as RBCs are sheered apart; endothelial damage in renal vessels → AKI). Do not give antibotics – increase risk of HUS!
Traveller's	**Most common** cause of diarrhoea after foreign travel **due to ETEC**

	(Enterotoxigenic *E. coli*)
Shigella spp.	**1-2 days incubation** → dysentery, tenesmus. Risk factor: MSM. Complications: **reactive arthritis, HUS, megacolon** (avoid anti-diarrhoeal meds).
Vibrio chlorae	Incubation 2-5 days → watery diarrhoea (rice water diarrhoea) **Tx:** electrolye replacement
Giardia	Faecal-oral spread of cysts (lake water). **Incubation of 1-3 weeks.** Persistent diarrhoea, flatulence, bloating, pain, malabsorptive Sx – **Sx last weeks to months.** Dx: stool microscopy (cysts and trophozoite = flagellated w 2 nuclei) ≥ 3 samples due to intermittent shedding. Cx: lactose intolerance. Tx: **metronidazole**
Cryptosporidium	Self-limiting diarrhoea in immunocompetent (contaminated water) but severe and chronic one in **immunosuppressed**. No clear Tx.
Entamoeba histolytica	Faecal-oral spread (cysts destroyed by boiling) Intestinal amoebiasis → insidious/relapsing colitis, appendicitis, toxic megacolon Invasive amoebiasis → liver abscess (anchovy sauce paste) = high swinging fevers, RUQ pain, LFT cholestatic picture. Dx: microscopy (cysts = many nuclei; trophozoite = no flagella, 1 nucleus) Tx: **metronidazole**

COELIAC DISEASE

- Pt: diarrhoea (steatorrhoea = stinky, floaty stools), weight loss, anaemia (B12, fol),
  neuropathy (B12 def).
- Other manifestations/complications: **dermatitis herpetiformis** = itchy crops of red
  vesicles in shins or elbows; **osteoporosis/osteopenia**; **hyposplenism** = offer yearly
  flu and 5-yearly pneumococcal vaccines; **rarely: GI T-cell lymphoma** (suspected if
  refractory Sx or persistent loss of weight) and **other GI cancers**.
- Dx: **anti-transglutaminase (anti-Ttg)** – this is an IgA antibody and in a considerable
  amount of coeliac patients, there is IgA deficiency – so IgA levels should be added;
  trial of gluten-free diet; duodenal Bx (gold-standard).
- Tx = gluten-free diet lifelong – can eat RICE, MAIZE, POTATOES, SOYA. **Avoid barley,
  rye, wheat, etc.**
- Dapsone may help with dermatitis herpetiformis

IRRITABLE BOWEL SYNDROME

- Rome criteria (Dx is from clinical Hx) – **recurrent abdo pain** average of 1 day per
  week, in the last 3 months, associated with **at least 2 of:**
  - Defecation related
  - Change in stool frequency
  - Change in stool form
  - And no red flags
- Tx:

- o Constipation-predominant IBS → water and fibre intake; bulk-forming laxatives e.g. macrogol or stimulant e.g. senna. **DO NOT use lactulose.**
- o Diarrhoea-predominant IBS → loperamide
- o Colic or bloating → anti-spasmodics e.g. mebeverine, hyoscine (avoid these in **paralytic ileus**)
- o Psych/visceral pain → super low-dose amitriptyline 10-20 mg
- o **Low FODMAP diet** (fermentable, poorly absorbed saccharides)

NUTRITIONAL DEFICIENCIES

- Vitamin B1 (thiamine)
  - o Wernicke encephalopathy: triad of confusion + ophthalmoplegia + ataxia. Korsakoff syndrome – confabulation, personality change, and permanent memory loss. Mamillary body damage.
  - o Dry beriberi – polyneuritis with muscle wasting
  - o Wet beriberi – high output HF (DCM) → oedema
- Vitamin B2 (riboflavin) → cheilosis of lips
- Vitamin B3 (niacin) → pellagra (Dermatitis, Diarrhoea, Dementia, Death)
  - o **Hartnup disease (AR)** – deficiency of Trp (renal tubular transporter defect) → unable to convert Trp to niacin → pellagra.
- Vitamin B6 (pyridoxine) → neuropathy, seizures, sideroblastic anaemia. S/E of isoniazid (should give B6 supplement)
- Vitamin B9 = folate → megaloblastic anaemia (see chapter on Haematology)
- Vitamin B12 = cobalamin → megaloblastic anaemia with subacute combined degeneration of cord (loss of proprioception and vibration sense = dorsal column; lateral corticospinal tracts = pyramidal/UMN signs + distal paraesthesia; spinocerebellar tracts = ataxia).
  - o **SACDC is one of few conditions that can cause a mixed LMN (absent DTR legs) and UMN (Positive Babinski) signs**
- Vitamin A, D, E, K are fat-soluble
  - o Vitamin A – night blindness, keratomalacia + sicca/xerophthalmia + Bitot spots (gray-whitish lesion on conjunctiva), immunosuppression, dry skin (xerosis)
  - o Vitamin D – decreased Ca/P, high PTH (secondary hyperparathyroidism), and high ALP from bone turnover. Rickets in children; **osteomalacia** in adults – presents as bony pain and muscle weakness.
  - o Vitamin E – haemolytic anaemia, skin manifestations (blisters), neurological presentation similar to SACDC (B12 deficiency)
  - o Vitamin K – clotting defects (protein C, S, factors 2, 7, 9, 10)
- Vitamin C (ascorbate) – scurvy (swollen gums + petechiae + poor wound healing)

HEPATOLOGY

Jaundice: an approach

Pre-hepatic	Hepatic	Post-hepatic (obstructive/cholestatic)
UCB ↑	UCB/CB ↑	CB ↑
So urobilinogen ↑ (NOT water sol)		So urobilinogen and sterocobilinogen ↓
So normal stools (a bit concentrated) Normal stools (a bit darker)	Dark urine Normal stools	**Dark urine** (from urine conj bilirubin - d pstick) **Pale stools + steatorrhea** (malabsorption) **Pruritus**
Pigmented bilirubin gallstones		ALP ↑ (biliary problem)
• **Haemolysis** (high levels of UCB overwhelm conjugating ability of liver) • Ineffective erythropoiesis (precursor destruction) • B12 deficiency	E.g. hepatitis, cirrhosis, drugs, Gilbert's	E.g. cholangitis, pancreatic CA, cholangioCA, parasites, liver flukes (*Clonorchis sinesis*), strictures

*UCB = unconjugated bilirubin, CB = conjugated bilirubin
** **Gilbert's syndrome**: unconjugated hyperbilirubinaemia = jaundice intermittently during times of stress (illness, fasting, exercise) due to lack of UGT-1A1 activity for conjugating bilirubin w glucuronate. There is no haemolysis, and is benign.

HEPATOTOXIC DRUGS:
Overdose of paracetamol, TB drugs (INH, rif, pyrazinamide), valproate, statins, Combined pill, MAO inhibitors, halothane anaesthetics.

- For liver function tests: use "ratios" not absolute numbers to show that either ALP or ALT is higher.
  - ALP 3X upper limit is acceptable. ALP is raised in **bone disease** (different isoform), smokers, Afro-Caribbean > Caucasians, children.
  - ALT 5X upper limit is acceptable. > 300 -> acute liver injury.
  - GGT helps differentiate between ALP from liver or bone disease.
- Hepatocellular pattern of damage and scenarios:
  - Alcoholic liver disease: AST > ALT. High bilirubin. Normal ALP. High GGT. Macrocytosis.
  - Fatty infiltration (NAFLD): mildly raised ALT (ALT > AST).
  - Ischaemic liver disease: ALT ++++, high LDH. Recognise signs of shock.
  - Drug-induced: ALT ++++
  - Acute viral hepatitis: ALT +++ & raised bilirubin.
  - Chronic viral hepatitis: ALT+
  - Autoimmune: ALT +++ in young woman of child-bearing age.
- Cholestatic pattern of injury
  - High ALP and GGT >> AST/ALT.
  - **Flucloxacillin gives a cholestatic picture**

- Causes of massively raised ALT (1000s): (1) acute viral hepatitis, (2) drug-induced (paracetamol)/toxins (deathcap mushrooms), (3) ischaemic liver disease e.g. Budd-Chiari syndrome, (4) autoimmune liver disease

Alcoholic hepatitis (MCC)
- Complications:
    - Eventual cirrhosis (end-stage liver damage)
        - Portal hypertension → ascites, splenomegaly, portosystemic shunts (oesophageal varices; caput medusa; rectal varices)
        - HCC risk
    - Delirium tremens and seizure risk on acute withdrawal (10-72 h)
        - DTs (= visual and tactile hallucinations + haemodynamic instability + confusion, tremors -> seizures). **Peak at day 3**.
        - Detox with chlordiazepoxide taper and thiamine cover (to prevent Wernicke encephalopathy + Korsakoff syndrome)
    - Malnutrition, peripheral neuropathy, macrocytic anaemia, dilated cardiomyopathy
- Consequences of liver failure
    - Failure of synthetic function – clotting, low alb, low oestrogen → upper GI bleed
    - Failure of metabolic function - hypoglycaemia, jaundice
    - Failure of toxin clearance → encephalopathy (NH3) + sepsis
    - Abnormal haemodynamics
        - **Diet:** low salt, fluid-restricted
        - **Spironolactone high dose** 100-400 mg OD (c.f. heart failure) + furosemide if fail.
        - **Paracentesis** (with human albumin solution replacement)
        - **Shunting** e.g. TIPS
        - Spontaneous bacterial peritonitis → fluid drained has high leucocytes (WCC > 300-500 million/L) or neutrophils > 250 million/L
            - *Common bugs: E. coli, klebsiella, Streptococci*
            - Tx (empirically) = **ceftriaxone IV**
            - PPx (high risk: low serum or ascitic alb, high INR) = **ciprofloxacin PO**
        - Hepato-renal syndrome
            - Stop diuretic, salt-poor albumin infusion to rehydrate, may need dialysis, TIPS, or transplant.
            - Avoid hypoK+
- **ACUTE LIVER FAILURE/DECOMPENSATION**
    - Triad of jaundice; upper GI bleed/coagulopathy; encephalopathy
    - AVOID
        - Constipative meds, sedatives, oral hypoglycaemics, normal saline (Na+), CYP450 inhibitors (enhance *warfarin* effect), hepatotoxics (paracetamol, MTX, isoniazid, azathioprine, oestrogen, 6-MP, aspirin, tetracyclins...)
    - **On encephalopathy:**

- Reduce nitrogen load (avoid constipation, upper GI bleed, transfusion, AKI = urea, infections, hypokalaemia)
- Tx: lactulose (is catabolised by gut flora to trap ammonia in gut)
- PPx: rifaximin (kills nitrogen forming gut flora)

- Cirrhosis grading: **CHILD-PUGH SCORE.**
  - Grade A = 5-6, grade C = 10-15. Score > 8 predicts variceal bleed risk.

Encephalopathy	None	Minimal (grade I –II)	Marked (grade III – IV)
Ascites	None	Slight	Moderate
Bilirubin (μmol/L)	< 34	34 – 51	> 51
PT (seconds more than normal)	1 – 3	4 – 6	> 6
Ascites	None	Slight	Moderate

Some facts on alcohol and alcoholism
- 14 units per week man or woman; do not binge – spread out.
- Unit calculation: ABV x ml
  - Pint (568 ml) of beer = 2 (3.6%) – 3 units (5.2%)
  - Glass of wine (175 ml) = 2 units (12%); small glass = 1.5 units (125 ml)
  - Shot (25 ml) of spirit = 1 unit (40%)
- CAGE (Cut down, Annoyed by criticism, Guilty, Eye-opener) – *suggestive* if > 2

Non-alcoholic fatty liver disease (2nd MCC)
- Suspect if liver disease developed in a patient who drink $\leq$ 18 units/week with risk factors: elderly, obese, dyslipidaemia, diabetic, and hypertensive/vasculopath.
- Dx: elastography USS (Fibroscan), biopsy
- Tx: address obesity and cardiovascular risk factors; avoid EtOH. **No drug of benefit.**

Viral hepatitis (3rd MCC)
- Hep A (2-6 weeks incubation: raised ALT only after 3 weeks+) → constitutional Sx and arthralgia. Faecal-oral route (shellfish) in Africa or South America + Mexico.
- Hep E – presents similarly to Hep A. Pigs, undercooked seafood, and contaminated water. India and China. **In pregnancy → high mortality** (fulminant hepatitis).
- Hep **B**
  - 1-6 months incubation;
  - DNA virus → blood products (haemophiliacs; HCW), IVDU (prisons), sex/direct contact
    - NEEDLE-STICK: **1 out of 3** if no vaccine (vs. hep C = 1 in 30, HIV 1 in 300). Post-exposure PPx:
      - Fully vaccinated + responder – HBV booster only

- Fully vaccinated + non-responder – HBV booster + HBIG
- 1-2 dose of vax – accelerated HBV + HBIG

Stage	LFTs	HBsAg (surface)	HBeAg ("e" antigen) and HBV DNA	HBcAb (core)	HBsAb
Acute	↑↑↑	+ (first to rise)	+	IgM	
Window	(↑)			IgM	
Resolved				IgG	IgG (protective)
Chronic	↑	+ (presence > 6 months defines chronic state)	+/- (presence of e antigen or HBV DNA indicates infectivity)	IgG	
Immunisation					IgG (protective)

Vaccine = surface antibodies to prevent virus from entering cells – so will never get core protein in people who are vaccinated. Core protein Ab implies <u>past</u> infection. PCR for monitoring therapy

- o Active immunisation: at-risk groups (as above) – 3 set (0, 1m, 6m)
  - Non-responders (<10 surface Ab) – give another 3 sets vaccination
  - Booster required (<100).
  - Otherwise retest 1y (100-1000) or 4y (>1000).
- o Treatment of active infection:
  - Interferon alpha 1st line → tenofovir 2nd line
- o Key associations: **Polyarteritis nodsa (HbsAg)**, membranous nephropathy
- **Hep C**
  - o RNA virus that spreads by blood. Chronic Cirrhosis → HCC.
  - o Anti-HCV = exposure, HCV PCR = ongoing/chronic
  - o Tx (newer drugs):
    - Sofosbuvir/ledipasvir – inhibitors
    - Ribavirin – nucleoside analogue.
  - o HIV co-infection common – requires ART.
  - o Key associations: **cryo-globulinaemia**, autoimmune hepatitis and other autoimmune disease (polymyositis, thyroiditis), porphyria

- Other infections affecting the liver: EBV, CMV, **malaria**, yellow fever, leptospirosis

Fitz-Hugh-Curtis syndrome
Liver capsule inflammation causing RUQ pain due to transabdominal spread of chlamydial or gonococcal infection, often with PID ± 'violin-string' adhesions

Autoimmune (4th MCC)

- Type 1 (commoner, 80%) – **anti-SMOOTH MUSCLE (SM)*** and sometimes ANA. Usual autoimmune stereotype.
  *Anti-SM not to be confused with Anti-Smith (anti-Sm), the antibody found in lupus.
- Type 2 (less common) – Europeans kids, progressive and less treatable. **LKM1** antibody +ve. No ANA.
- No lab test is pathognomonic (Dx of exclusion) – LFTs, **hyperIgG**, auto-antibod es as above, **absence of other causes** (e.g. negative viral serology)
- Tx: steroids → AZA, ciclosporin → liver transplant.

Budd-Chiari syndrome

- Infraction of liver secondary to **heaptic vein** obstruction → massively raised ALT
- Acutely PAINFUL hepatomegaly, ascites, abdominal pain, and in cardiovascular shock
- Risk factors: HCC (invasion into hepatic vein + prothrombogenic); *steroids*
- Tx: surgery (100% mortality if not treated)

PBC vs PSC

Primary biliary cholangitis	Primary sclerosing cholangitis
• Autoimmune *granulomatous* destruction of intrahepatic bile duct	• Fibrotic (strictures) of **intra AND extra**hepatic ducts
• Mid-aged women, who itches and tires (obstructive jaundice)	• Mid-aged men with IBD
• Malabsorption	• Malabsorption
• **Anti-mitochondrial Ab**	• Histology: periductal fibrosis w onion-skin appearance
• ALP +++, cholesterol +++ → xanthomas	• MRCP: beaded appearance
• Autoimmune begets autoimmune	• **P-ANCA**
• Cirrhosis and HCC	• ALP +++
	• **High risk cholangiocarcinoma** (screen); cirrhosis and HCC

Genetic liver disease
- Wilson's – *ATP7B* ATPase mutation (AR) → lack of copper transport = accumulation:
  - Liver → cirrhosis, hepatomegaly → HCC eventually
  - CNS (LATE stage) → movement disorders (basal ganglia degeneration) + cognitive decline (subcortical: slow to solve problems); depression ☹
  - Eyes → Kayser-Fleischer ring (Descemet's membrane).
  - Arthritis, grey skin, blue nails
  - Haemolysis
  - **Dx:** 24 hour urinary excretion, moderately raised LFTs, serum copper and caeruloplasmin **LOW**, biopsy and gene testing.
  - **Tx:** lifelong penicillamine *if no CNS Sx* (S/E: drug-induced lupus, nephrotic syndrome, and pancytopenia → monitor FBC, copper + protein urinary excretion); liver transplant.
  - Diet: avoid high copper (liver, chocolate, nuts, mushroom, shellfish)
- Haemochromatosis – Celtic ancestry (*HFE* mutations – increased intestinal iron absorption). Accumulation of iron in body:
  - Arthritis + pseudogout of knee (chondrocalcinosis)
  - Slate-grey pigmentation
  - Chronic liver disease → HCC eventually
  - Dilated cardiomyopathy
  - Insulin-dependent diabetes (deposition in pancreas)
  - Hypogonadism (testicular atrophy due to *pituitary* gland dysfunction)
  - **Dx: high ferritin** and **ferritin saturations** in context of low inflammatory markers (ferritin is an acute phase reactant); moderately raised LFTs. Liver Bx with Perl's/Prussian blue stain.
  - **Tx:** regular venesection; chelators: desferrioxamine
  - **Diet:** avoid Fe-rich foods (Indian Balti curries – cast iron cookware; liver); uncooked marine fish (contains bacteria that thrive on high plasma Fe); EtOH.
- A1AT deficiency
  - Combination of emphysema and cholestatic jaundice should raise suspicion
  - Usually, serine protease inhibitor usually controls inflammatory cascade.
  - Made in liver → mutations = unable to transport proteins out = accumulate.
  - Genetics – variants based on electrophoresis: **M**edium (60% produced), **S**low, **Z** (very slow – 15% produced). PiMM = normal genotype; PiZZ = high risk
  - Dx: **low** A1AT levels, **obstructive** pattern of spirometry, liver Bx, genotyping
  - Tx: *smoking cessation, vaccines, pooled IV A1AT from human plasma, lung and liver transplant.*

Liver masses in summary:
- Malignancy
  - MCC: mets (breast, bronchus, gut/stomach, uterus)
  - HCC – causes: hepatitis B (worldwide leading cause), hep C, cirrhosis, NAFLD, anabolic steroids, aflatoxin (*Aspergillus*)
- Benign masses
  - MCC: haemangioma – incidental. Do not biopsy as it will bleed.
  - Adenomas – associated with anabolic steroids (weightlifters), COCP and pregnancy (oestrogen).

> **GENERAL TIPS**
> - Interpretation of anaemia screen is a test favourite
>
> - It is worthwhile to know the presentation of various leukaemia and lymphoma based on patient's characteristic (e.g. age, B symptoms)
>
> - Another high-yield topic examiners like to go after are the clotting defects

6. HAEMATOLOGY

ANAEMIA

Microcytic anaemia
- Iron deficiency
  - Hb low, MCV low, MCH low
  - Haematinics: serum Fe low, ferritin low, **transferrin high**
  - Things to rule out: coeliac disease and bowel cancer
  - Tx: Fe supplementation (S/E: constipation, black stools); IV iron if oral not possible or in **CKD**.
- Thalassaemia
  - ALPHA
    - Gene deletion (1 = minima, 2 = minor, 3 = HbH disease, 4 = Barts)
    - Cis deletions in Asians → therefore risk hydrops baby
    - **HbH** disease:
      - **Beta chain form tetramer β4 = HbH**, damaging RBC membrane → haemolytic anaemia (occurs straight after birth when body tries to switch from HbF to HbA/A2)
      - **Dx: HPLC/electrophoresis**
      - **Tx:** iron transfusion, splenectomy

NORMAL Hb

- $HbF = \alpha2\gamma2$

- $HbA = \alpha2\beta2$

- $HbA_2 = \alpha2\delta2$

	Hb	MCV	RDW
αα/αα	Normal	Normal	Normal
αα/α−	Low	Low	Normal
αα/−− or α−/α−	Low	Low	Raised
α−/−−	VERY low	VERY low	VERY raised

- o BETA thal
  - Gene MUTATIONS. African or Mediterranean.
  - 2 beta genes on Ch 11 → mutations lead to absent ($\beta 0$) or diminished ($\beta 1/+$)
  - Minor = β / $\beta 1$ or β / $\beta 0$ = **microcytic, hypochromic RBC with target cells** (similar to Fe deficiency **BUT** thal's MCV is too low for the Hb)
    - HPLC/electrophoresis = *slightly less HbA, slight rise HbA2 (>3.5%) = hallmark*
  - Intermedia = β 0/ $\beta 0$ = a
    - HPLC/electrophoresis = HbA halved, rise of HbF >> HbA2 (hallmark)
  - Major = β 0/ $\beta 0$ = Cooley's anaemia → unpaired alpha chain tetramerise causing damage to RBC → ineffective erythropoiesis → extramedullary haematopoiesis (hepatosplenomegaly, frontal bossing, crew-cut skull, chipmunk facies)
    - HPLC/electrophoresis = presence of HbF with **no** HbA and some HbA2 = *hallmark*
  - Tx: folate supplement (turnover high), chronic transfusion with desferroxamine chelation, GH Tx for endocrine complications (DM, hypothyroid), ascorbate to remove Fe in urine, bone marrow transplant is curative.
  - **Cx:** at risk of aplastic crisis if parvovirus B19 infection; *osteopenia* (zoledronate supplementation)

Anaemia of chronic disease

- Can be micro (late) or normocytic (initial), **LOW transferrin is the key differentiator**
- Due to poor usage of iron for erythropoiesis = "functional" iron deficiency (chronic inflammation → hepcidin produced by liver → sequestering iron in macrophage stores)
- Tx underlying cause – exogenous EPO in subset (cancer, CKD). Iron supplement not effective unless IV iron to overcome "functional" iron deficiency.

Macrocytic anaemia

- **Folate** deficiency
  - o **Causes:** Poor diet (folate in "foilage" = green vegetables + fruits, liver, nuts) or increased demand (pregnancy, renal failure on dialysis, liver disease, heart failure) or inhibited (antifolates e.g. MTX, phenytoin, EtOH) or malabsorption (absorbed by duodenum and proximal jejunum → resection; coeliac disease)
  - o Last 4 months (minimal stores)
  - o FBC: **megaloblastic** anaemia with **hypersegmented** Nø; serum folate low; B12 <->
  - o **Tx:** folate replacement 5 mg/day 4 months **with B12** (to avoid precipitation of subacute combined degeneration of cord, if B12 levels low)

- o **PPx:** pregnancy, long-term MTX usage.
- **B12 deficiency**
  - o Last longer so rare (4 years storage in liver)
  - o Dietary cause rare (unless pure vegan, as B12 = <u>animal origin</u>)
  - o Other causes: defect in processing pathway or malabsorption (cleaved by HCl in stomach; bind intrinsic factor (produced from parietal cells) → complex is absorbed in **ileum)**
    - **PERNICIOUS anaemia** (MCC UK)
      - **AUTOIMMUNE** destruction of parietal cells.
      - **Autoimmune begets autoimmune** → signs of vtilligo, hypothyroid (Hashimoto's)
      - **Anti-parietal cells more sensitive**/less specific
      - **Anti-IF more specific**/less sensitive
      - Increased risk of gastric cancer
    - Gastric bypass, terminal ileitis of Crohn's, pancreatic insufficiency
  - o **B12 deficiency signs and symptoms:**
    - Beefy red tongue (glossitis) + angular stomatitis
    - Sensory polyneuropathy
    - Cognitive impairment
    - Optic atrophy (nutritional)
    - SACD (symmetrical dorsal column, distal sensory, wide gait),
    - Osteoporosis.
  - o **LABS: megaloblastic** anaemia with **hypersegmented** Nø; serum folate <->; B12 low. High homocysteine (thrombosis risk, same as folate); high MMA (c.f. folate def).
  - o **Tx: B12 replacement** (hydroxycobalamin 1mg IM alternate days 2 weeks then 1 mg every 3 months for life); Fe can accelerate Tx
  - o **Beware:** hypokalaemia from transcellular shift as K+ taken up by newly formed haematopoietic cells (replace K+ with treatment)
- **Other causes of macrocytosis:** EtOH, hypothyroidism, drug-induced (anti-folates, cytotoxics e.g. 5-FU, ART for HIV, hydroxyurea), myelodysplastic syndromes, reticulocytosis e.g. in haemolysis

Haemolytic Anaemia

Normocytic anaemia – 2 main mechanisms: haemolysis or underproduction.

Haemolysis compensated by raised reticulocyte count (RC). Reticulocytes are young RBCs released from marrow and have bluish cytoplasm due to basophilic residual RNA. Normal count is 1-2% and roughly 1-2% RBCs (lifespan – 120 days) are removed each day to be replaced by reticulocytes.

RC is **falsely elevated in anaemia** because it is measured as a total %RBC (so fall in RBC = rise RC). Hence it is often *corrected* by the lab (RC x HCT/45).

Corrected RC of < 3% indicates underproduction.

Intravascular haemolysis	Extravascular haemolysis
RBC destroyed by reticuloendothelial system (macrophages of spleen, liver, LN)	RBCs broken down within vessels
Haem broken down into Fe (which is recycled) and protoporphyrinogen (⬚ broken down to unconjugated bilirubin; carried by albumin ⬚ delivered to liver for conjugation and excreted through bile) Low haptoglobin High unconjugated bilirubin (prehepatic jaundice) → predisposes GS High RC (> 3%; marrow hyperplasia) High LDH	Haemoglobinaemia (Hb released into blood) Low haptoglobin + haemoglobinuria (haptoglobin no longer handle load) Haemosiderinuria (renal tubular cells picked some filtered Hb up which is broken down to Fe and accumulate as haemosiderin; these tubular cells eventually shed off). High unconjugated bilirubin (prehepatic jaundice) → predisposes GS High RC (> 3%; marrow hyperplasia) High LDH

- **Hereditary spherocytosis (AD)** – less deformable RBCs (spherocytes) prone to haemolysis → mild haemolytic anaemia, high unconjugated bilirubin. Tests: osmotic fragility (old), SDS-PAGE. **Tx:** folate supplementation, splenectomy. **Cx:** B19 crisis.
- **Sickle cell disease** – AR mutations of β chain of Hb. Protective against malaria (African descent).
  - SC trait = 1 mutated, 1 normal gene
    - 40-50% HbS in RBCs, 55% HbA, 2% HbA_2
  - SCD occurs when **2 chains are abnormal:**
    - 90% HbS in RBCs, 8% HbF, 2% HbA_2 (no HbA)
    - Polymerisation in conditions of hypoxaemia (flights), dehydration, acidosis
    - **Hydroxyurea** increases HbF and is used during sickle cell crisis.
    - Cells continue to sickle and de-sickle while passing microcirculation, these are fragile– leading to haemolysis.

- Extravascular haemolysis w SiSx as above
- Intravasuclar haemolysis w decreased haptoglobin and *target cells* on smear
- Massive *extramedullary haematopoiesis/hyperplasia*
- Facial bones and skulls (similar to thalasseamia)
- Hepatomegaly (NOT splenomegaly because the spleen is autoinfarcted)
- B19 aplastic crisis risk.

- Furthermore, extensive sickling leads to vaso-occlusive crisis *anywhere* in micro-circulation. **PPt: cold, hypoxia, dehydration, infection.**

  Acutely:

  - Dactylitis – swollen fingers or toes; hands and feets are affected if < 3 y – due to vaso-occlusive infarcts in bones.
  - Avascular necrosis e.g., of femoral head
  - Acute chest syndrome – vaso-occlusion in pulmonary microcirculation
    - Pt: T°, chest pain, SOB, wheeze, cough, and tachypnoea with a **prodrome of pain** 2.5 days before any abnormalities in CXR in (50% patient)
    - Path: pulmonary infiltrates involving complete lung segments.
    - Incidence: 0.1 episodes/patient/year
    - Aetiology of infiltrates: PNA (chief cause are: *Mycoplasma*, viruses, *Chlamydia*); also: **fat embolism** from marrow or infection
    - Vichinsky study ◻ 11% need ventilation (i.e. progressed to type **2** RF), 13% have CNS Sx, 9% of > 20y die.
    - MCC death in adult patients
    - **Chronic Cx:** fibrosis → PHTN → cor pulmonale
    - **Tx: bronchodilators, empirical Abx, transfusion, ITU for ventilation, exchange transfusion**
  - Renal papillary necrosis – pt: gross haematuria and proteinuria → **Chronic Cx:** CKD
  - Pain crisis → **PCA morphine**
  - CNS infarction = stroke, seizures, cognitive defect
  - Low-flow priapism (DDx: CML) → Tx: **alpha agonist or blood aspiration or irrigation with saline.**
  - **GENERAL Tx of vaso-occlusive crises:** ANALGESIA, IV fluids, transfusion may be needed to reduce HbSS, hydroxyurea,

exchange transfusion if rapidly worsening (chest crisis, CNS event, MSOF)
- Chronically:
  - **Auto-splenectomy/infarction** – shrunken and fibrotic spleen
    - Increased risk of infection w encapsulated organisms e.g. pneumococci, meningococcus, and *Hib*.
    - Affected children should be vaccinated by 5y (MCC death in children: 40%)
    - **Increases risk of *non-typhoidal Salmonella* osteomyelitis**
    - Howell-Jolly bodies appear on film
  - Sickle cell retinopathy
    - Crystallised Hb damages and occludes the vessels of eye
    - Can be non-proliferative due to v-o + local ischaemia ("salmon patches" = oval shapes = haemorrhage from superficial vessels) – mainly **HbSS**. PPx: hydroxyurea
    - And proliferative (usually in **HbSC** and **HbSThal** disease) ☐ <u>chronic</u> localised v-o = upregulation of VEGF → new proliferation → vitreous haemorrhage and tractional RD.
      - Tx: anti-VEGF, lasers, or surgical.
- Sequestration crisis: MAINLY in children because adult spleens are atrophic
  - Refers to pooling of blood in spleen ± liver ☐ organomegaly + severe anaemia + shock
  - Tx: urgent transfusion

- **Tests (SCD):** normocytic anaemia + sickle w target cells on film + Howell-Jolly bodies; high bilirubin; HPLC/electrophoresis; PCR

- Tx: hydroxyurea (reduce *f* of crisis), immunisation (pneumococcal, meningococcal) + PPx Abx (pen V) & rescue Abx (cef in children/repeated admission); folate supplement; transfusions; stroke prevention (if Fe overloaded). BONE MARROW TRANSPLANT curative but limited.

	HbSS	HbSA (SCT/carrier)	HbSA/α -thal	HbS/ β° thal	HbS/β⁺ thal
HbA	NONE	55% (> 50%)	70%	15%	25% (< 50%) Milder because have 5-15% beta globin in Hb
HbS	90%	40% (< 50%) *If < 40% = also alpha thal trait	25% (< 40%*)	65%	55% (> 50%)
HbA₂	2%	2%	3%	5%	3%
HbF	8%	3%	2%	15%	20%
Film	Hb, MCV, MCH, and MCHC ↔		Microcytic anaemia		

Table summarizing HPLC/electrophoresis results in haemoglobinopathies

- **G6PD deficiency** – XLR disease where Glucose-6-phosphate dehydrogenase is reduced → RBC now prone to oxidative stress as GSH not regenerated
  - **PPt:** drugs = SULFA (aspirin, sulphonamide, quinine including tonic water, dapsone); Fava beans; Henna tattoo; infections and illnesses
  - **Pt:** attacks within hours (rapid) → anaemia + jaundice w haemaglobinuria and flank pain (Hb is nephrotoxic)
  - **Film:** Heinz bodies (= precipitated Hb), bite cells (splenic MØ removed Heinz bodies)
  - **Screen:** enzyme assay
  - **Tx:** self-limiting, transfusion if severe
- **Autoimmune haemolytic anaemia (AIHA)**
  - Ig directed RBC destruction, mediated by macrophages
  - Tests: **DIRECT** Coomb's/antiglobulin test (DCT or DAT) to detect RBC already coated with antibodies (agglutinate with anti-IgG)
  - IgG disease = WARM agglutinin = extravascular, central body (warmer); more associated with autoimmune disease (SLE), also CLL, haptens (penicillin, cephalosporin), methyldopa, quinidine. **Tx:** treat underlying cause; steroids; IVIg to distract macrophages. Splenectomy as last resort.
  - IgM disease = COLD agglutinin = intravascular, peripheries (colder) → acrocyanosis. Associated with EBV, HIV, and mycoplasma

Porphyria
- Acute intermittent porphyria: 20-40 ys → 6 Ps
  - Porphobilinogen deaminase defect (AD) → d-ALA + porphobilinogen accumulation
  - Painful abdomen
  - Port-wine urine on sunlight exposure
  - Polyneuropathy
  - Psych disturbances e.g. depression
  - Ppt by drugs (P450 inducers, EtOH, starvation)
  - Tx: glucose and heme → inhibit ALA synthase → less d-ALA accumulation
- Porphyria cutanea tarda
  - Uroporphyrinogen decarboxylase defect (AD) in 1/3
  - 2/3 Others:
    - Liver (alcohol, hep B/C, haemochromatosis) - EtOH worsens it
    - OCT/HRT/dialysis
    - Rarely SLE, HIV
  - Pt: photosensitive blistering milia that is slow to heal, heal with hyperpigmentation
  - Tests: uroporphyrinogen, pink fluorescence of urine under Wood's lamp, ferritin
  - Tx chloroquine + venesection (if ferritin >600)

Transfusions
- **Platelets:** Stored at room temperature –bacteria contamination
  - **Active bleeding start**: <$30x10^9$ clinically significant bleeding, <$100x10^9$ if severe/CNS
  - **Prophylactic surgery aim**: >$50x10^9$ most 50-75x10^9 high risk >$100x10^9$ at critical site
  - **If no active bleeding start**: $10x10^9$ UNLESS (TTP, HIT, chronic BM failure, ITP)
- **Blood:** leukodepletion, plasma derivatives fractionated from imported plasma, since 2004 received blood can't donate
  - CMV neg – **granulocyte, intrauterine, neonates up to 28d post expected date of delivery**, pregnancy
  - Irradiated – **old**, BM/stem cell transplant, immunocompromised, Hodgkin's (inc previous)
  - Washed – recurrent/severe reactions to red cells, or IgA deficient patients with anti IgA Ab
- **FFP** – clinically significant w/o major haemorrhage with PT or APTT >1.5, universal donor is AB blood (no anti-A/B)
- **Cryoprecipitate** - clinically significant w/o major haemorrhage + fibrinogen <1.5g/L, in DIC, liver failure, vWD, invasive surgery, contains: F8, vWF, fibrinogen, F13, from further processing FFP, much smaller volume (15ml cf 150ml)

- **Prothrombin complex concentrate** – emergency reversal in severe bleeding or head injury with suspected ICH, or prophylaxis in emergency surgery, contains: F2, 9, 10 (some have 7)
- **Reactions:**
    - **Non-immune mediated** – hypocalcaemia, CCF, infections, hyperkalaemia
    - **Acute**
        - Nonhaemolytic febrile reaction (2% RBC 30% platelet WBC HLA Ab vs fragment and cytokines leak during storage) – rx slow/stop + paracetamol
        - Minor allergic (urticaria/itch from foreign plasma protein) -temporary stop + antihistamine
        - Anaphylaxis (IgA def with anti IgA ab <u>mostly from IgM</u>) – rx stop, im adrenaline
        - Acute haemolytic reaction (fever/abdo pain/hypotension from ABO incompatible) – rx stop, IVF, direct Coombs, repeat cross match
        - TACO (pulm oedema, HTN 6h) – rx slow/stop, furosemide
        - TRALI (hypoxia, CXR pulm infiltrates, fever, hypotension 6h) rx stop, o2
    - **Chronic:** delayed haemolytic reaction (5-10d, Ab to Rh) anaphylaxis
    - **GVHD** – from T cell (donor) vs tissues, we try and stop with ciclosporin
        - Acute (100d) – skin, GI, liver
        - Chronic (>100d) – dry eyes, skin changes, CLD, weight loss

WHITE CELL DISORDERS

Myeloproliferative
- **CML** (Philadelphia t9;22, so NOT JAK2/CALR/MPL)
    - Maturing granulocytes, fatigue, weight loss, night sweats, priapism, tinnitus
    - Ix – **FISH/karyotype/PCR**, 50-400 WBC++ can see high platelets, low Hb, <10% blasts, BM hypercellular
    - Prognosis – chronic → accelerated → blast crisis (ALL/AML)
    - Rx – **imatinib (TKI)**, hydroxycarbamide sometimes
- **PV** (JAK2 95%)
    - Viscosity headache, dizzy, stroke, pruritis (hot bath), ruddy complection, thrombosis, bleeding, plethora, HSM, erythromelalgia, 20% gouty arthritis, peptic ulcer can lead to <u>fibrosis</u> (secondary MF), secondary PV can be caused by altitude, RCC, VHL, PKD, COPD, heart disease
    - 15% MF
    - Ix – **Flow Cytometry**, high Hb, 50% increased platelets, low EPO, low neutrophil
    - Rx – **venesection**, low dose aspirin, hydroxycarbamide (slight % secondary leukaemia)
- **MF**
    - Lethargy, HSM, weight loss, night sweats, fever, pallor, more uric acid
    - Ix – teardrop cells, **BM fibrosis**, high platelets and WBC, <u>dry tap BM</u>, high urate & LDHH (high cell turnover)
    - Rx – hydroxycarbamide, thalidomide
- **ET**
    - <u>Thrombosis/bleeding</u> – <u>digital</u> ischaemia, stroke, Budd-Chiari
    - Ix – 50% JAK2, no criteria for other MP, >500 platelets, 20% calreticulin (CALR)
    - Rx – <u>alpha-interferon</u> (women childbearing), <u>hydroxycarbamide</u>, low dose aspirirn, anagrelide

Leukaemia
- Leukaemoid reaction – severe infection/haemolysis/haemorrhage/metastatic cancer – high LALP, Dohle bodies (toxic granulation), left shift of neutrophils
- <u>AML</u>: Down's (M7), radiation, benzene, good mutations are t(15;17), Bad is trisomy, FAB classification M0-7, just need to know M3:
    - **APML** (promyelocytic M3 10%) – granules, can cause DIC and can be treated **all-trans retinoic acid**.
    - **Symptoms**: BM failure: pallor, tiredness, exertional SOB, infection, bleeding, infiltrate gums in M5
    - **Ix:** low platelets, >blast 20%, auer rods, immunophenotyping
    - **Rx:** CTX (80% remission), platelet/RBC transfusion or BMT (RIC-MUD)
- <u>ALL (B-ALL more common or T-ALL)</u>, 80% childhood leukaemia2-4y, weak, bruising, otitis, media/infection, bone pain, enlarged LN, headache,

- o Poor: FAB L3 type, T/B cell surface marker, Philadelphia t9;22, age <2 cr >10, male, CNS involvement, high initial WBC >100, non-Caucasian, hypodiploidy
  - o Good: FAB L1 type, common ALL, pre-B-ALL, low initial WBC, del9p, t(12;21), t(1;19)
  - o **Rx** – 4 phase chemotherapy
- CLL (99% B-cell clonal), >50y, often asymptomatic, constitutional (anorexia, weight loss), 10% **warm AIHA, immune thrombocytopenia** (bleed), **hypogammaglobulinaemia** (infections), red cell aplasia, angioedema (vs C1 esterase), **3% Richter's transformation to LARGE CELL**, SLL lymphoma in BM/LN
  - o Prognosis – Poor: male, >70y, lymphocyte >50, prolymphocyte >10%, doubling <12m, raised LDH, CD38+, TP53, del17p, Good: del13q (most common, 50%)
  - o Blood film – lymphocytes, smear/smudge cells
  - o Rx – watch and wait, high WCC not indication to treat, consider when other counts start to fall or B symptoms: fludarabine, ciclosporin, rituximab (=CR), ibrutinib if failed previous
  - o HAIRY CELL – subtype: Pancytopenia, splenomegaly, skin vasculitis, dry tap BM, TRAP stain positive, Rx CTX (cladribine, pentostatin), immunotherapy (rituximab, INF-alpha)
- Myelodysplastic, Low 2 cell lines, BM has abnormal HPSC, elderly, anaemia, 30% AML, **Rx:** supportive (CTX not great)

Lymphoma

If LN >1cm present for >6 weeks, need investigation: excision biopsy (**Biopsy → then Stage Ann-Arbor Score)**

1. Single group
2. 2+ on one side of diaphragm
3. Both sides of diaphragm
4. Extralymphatic (BM/liver)

Hodgkin's lymphoma

- 15-35 or >60 (bimodal), RARE, CD20, Reed Sternberg, 30% EBV+, 4 histology
- 4 histology: Nodular sclerosing (70%; women, lacunar cells), mixed cellularity (20%; lots R-S cell), lymphocyte predominant (5%), lymphocyte depleted (rare)
- CD30, EtOH induced pain, cough (intrathoracic disease), Pel-Ebstein fever
- Worse prognosis if B symptoms (loss >10% 6 mo), poor age >45, stage IV, Hb <10.5, male, albumin <40, WBC >15Rx – external beam radiation therapy, brentuximab, ABVD chemo

Others (high grade DLBCL, BL, CTCL, low grade FL, WM)

- Lymphoid line (ALL) → pre B → immature (Burkitt's) → before Ag (CLL) →Afte⁻ Ag (MCL, FL) → activated (DLBCL) → plasma (Waldenstrom/Myeloma)
- **Waldenstrom macroglobulinaemia** (mature IgM), >50y, headache, HSM, visual disturbance, cold agglutins, anaemia, hyperviscosity, Raynauld rx exchange/cido
- **Follicular lymphoma** (t14;18), BCL-2 increase, LN, BM, liver, GI, skin, 30% LCL, rx CVP + rituximab

- **Mantle cell** (t11;14 CD5+ve),cyclin D1 and heavy chain Ig, 60y, widespread LN/liver/BM/GI, aggressive & poor prognosis, rx ritux
- **Marginal zone** – extranode, gastric MALT (h. pylori), thyroid, saliva, lungs, spleen
- **Diffuse large B cell** – 40% lymphoma, fast, common HNL, high grade, sweats, fever, GI, testis, bone, rx CHOP + ritux
- **Burkitt** (t(8:14) MYC on ch8), starry sky (lymphocyte + macrophage with dead apoptotic tumour cells), 3 types: endemic (EBV), sporadic (old, frail), immunodeficiency (HIV), rx CODOX-M/IVAC, >90% cure rate

Myeloma
- Older patients. Part of paraproteinaemia spectrum (MGUS, MGRS, smoldering, and full-blown MM)
- Present: **CRAB symptoms** - do a myeloma screen fo any new AKI in older patients
    - Calcium (high) → bones, stones, groans, psych overtones + anorexia
    - Renal failure (multifactorial... cast nephropathy, light chain disease, amyloidosis, pre-renal AKI, hyperCa2+, NSAIDs for bone pain, cryoglobulinaemia)
    - Anaemia (from bone marrow failure... also other -penias = bleeding
    - Bone pain (L spine), compression # vertebra (activate osteoclasts = LYTIC lesion)
    - Others: amyloidosis → peripheral neuropathy, macroglossia, cardiomegaly, carpal tunnel; hyperviscosity (IgA); and encapsulated bacteria infection (PNA and sinusitis)
- Labs:
    - Film – Roleaux formation, anaemia (normocytic, normochromic)
    - Raised ESR, AKI, hypercalcaemia
    - SPEP – M-spike (IgG, IgA)
    - UPEP – 10% no M-spike... so look for Bence-Jones protein (free light chain κ/λ)
    - Serum free light chain – disproportionately relatively high κ or λ level
    - Bx and other scans (CT-PET/MRI for bony involvement)
- Treatment:
    - High Ca2+ → IVF, bisphosphonates,
    - Anaemia → EPO
    - Plasma exchange, dialysis
    - Chemo: bortezonib) or radio (bone pain)
    - Autograft stem cell therapy

CLOTTING DISORDERS

Clotting factors and labs
- APTT = 12, 11, 9, 8, 10, 5, 2, 1 (intrinsic)
- PT = 7, 10, 5, 2, 1 (more sensitive – FVII has shorter t1/2)
- Thrombin time = if heparin or fibrinogen deficiency
- Clotting in arterial system mostly platelet driven (when in contact with endothelium/atheroma), in venous system is due to blood stasis so clotting factor driven
- LMWH monitoring – factor Xa level

Thrombocytopenia
- **Idiopathic thrombocytopenic purpura (ITP)**
  - **Primary:** IgG antibodies against platelet antigens such as GpIIb/IIIa (**XLR**)
  - Secondary causes: SLE, leukaemia, quinine, heparin, HIV, hep C, antiphospholipid syndrome
  - Evans syndrome – ITP + AIHA
  - **Acute form in kids:** 2 weeks after viral infection → self-limiting
  - **Chronic form in adults:** women of childbearing age. Pt: fluctuating course of purpura at pressure sites, **nosebleed, menorrhagia**. NO splenomegaly
    - Labs: no single best test – Dx of exclusion (low platelet + normal coagulation PT/PTT)
    - Tx: steroids + IVIg ± splenectomy or rituximab in refractory cases
    - Avoid platelet transfusion (will get destroyed) if possible
- **Thrombotic thrombocytopenic Purpura (TTP)** – decreased ADAMTS13 = cannot cleave von Willebrand factor into monomer = multimer accumulation = platelet microthrombi → shearing RBC as it passes through vessels (microangiopathyic haemolytic anaemia, MAHA)
  - **Labs:** low platelet (consumed), haemolytic anaemia (DCT negative as not autoimmune) with schistocytes
  - **Pt:** MORE neurology (than HUS), AKI + haematuria (less than HUS), fever
  - Tx: STEROIDS and plasma exchange; rituximab,
  - AVOID: platelet transfusion (will be consumed and make things worse).
- **Haemolytic Uraemic Syndrome (HUS)** – MCC AKI in children: 90% infection (O157:H7), 10% atypical.
  - **Pt:** profuse diarrhoea -> bloody 1-3 d later, abdo pain, vomiting, fever. Stool sample for phage typing;
  - Labs: same as above
  - Tx: supportive +/- dialysis
- **Heparin-induced Thrombocytopenia (HIT)** – Ab against platelet factor 4 and heparin complex → platelet activation, 5-10 days after heparin given → 50% reduction in platelets, thrombosis, skin allergy,
- **Disseminated intravascular coagulopathy (DIC)** – thrombosis yet bleed from every orifices due to consumptive coagulopathy (microthrombi = MAHA, infarction)
  - **Labs:** low plt, high APTT/PT/thrombin, low fibrinogen

- o **Tx**: platelet replacement, cryoprecipitate (fibrogen + FVIII + FXIII + vWF), FFP (coagulation factors), blood transfusion

Thrombophilia
- Presents as thrombosis – DVT, strokes, sinus venous thrombosis, PE, Budd-Chiari, MI
- In order of prevalence:
  - o Factor V Leiden (Activated protein C resistance)
  - o Prothrombin 20210A gene mutation
  - o Protein C def (AD)
  - o Protein S def (AD)
  - o Antithrombin III
- **Acquired drug causes:** tamoxifen, olanzapine, HRT, OCP (stop OCP 4 weeks before elective op).

Haemophilia
- Von Willebrand disease:
  - o Mainly AD
  - o vWF promotes platelet adhesion to damaged endothelium, and stabilises FVIII
  - o Type 1 disease – partial deficiency of factor (80%)
  - o Type 2 disease – abnormal form
  - o Type 3 disease – total lack of factor (AR)
  - o **Pt:** MILD mucosal or skin bleeding (superficial)
  - o Tests: **APTT high (as FVIII decreased)** but PT normal; **bleeding time increased** (platelets affected); **Ristocetin test** (induces agglutination of platelet by causing vWF to bind GpIb… however in vWD this does not happen)
  - o Tx: nasal, SC, or IV desmopressin (ADH analogue binds V2R = increase vWF release from endothelial cells).
- Haemophilia
  - o X-linked recessive → **MALES**
  - o A = lack factor 8
  - o B = lack factor 9, 'Christmas Disease'
  - o **DEEP TISSUE bleeding:** hemarthroses & hematomas
  - o Tests: **prolonged APTT** only.
  - o Tx: minor – elevation, pressure, TXA
    - ▪ Severe → recombinant FVIII/FIX (15% develop antibodies to it)

Heparin
- **Unfractionated** (Xa + IIa) – inhibit Xa, IXa, XIa, XIIa give by continuous IV infusion, requires monitoring by **APTT** to 1.5-2.5 (difficult)
- **Fondaparinux** (bind ATIII Xa) – lower HIT rate
- **LMWH** (bind ATIII Xa) – s/c renal excreted, easy dosing, t1/2 10h (longer), no monitoring
- Protamine sulphate reversal (UFN full, LMWH partial, fondaparinux no)
- Side effects: long term osteoporosis, pain on injection site, hyperkalaemia (inhibition of aldosterone secretion)

DOAC
- NOT for metal heart valves, arterial thrombosis, pregnancy, breastfeeding
- USE for non-valvular AF (not significant MS/metal valve), VTE
- *Eliminated routes: dabigatran (renal), rivaroxaban (liver), apixaban (faecal)*
- *Interactions – AED, anti-retroviral, anti-fungals, rifampicin*
- Vs thrombin (dab), vs Xa (others)
- For VTE – now use apixaban 1st line: dab/edox needs 5d heparin, dabigatran can cause GI bleeds, increased menorrhagia in rivaroxaban
- Coagulation test – need to do a specific assay, APTT/PT not specific, only **thrombin time** for dab
- Bleeding: IV TXA + Give **PCC** (run plasma through machine, just give) e.g. BERIPLEX, give **oral charcoal** if taken <4h ago. **No specific antidotes except: dabigatran – can use Idarucizumab.**

Warfarin
- Reduces II, VII, IX and X and protein C
- VTE – aim 2.5, if recurrent/PE 3.5, AF – target INR 2.5, Mechanical heart valves depends on location, age, 2.5-3.5 in old, 2-3 in new
- **Side effects**: haemorrhage, teratogenic (though can be used in breastfeeding), skin necrosis (reduce biosynthesis of vitamin C → thrombosis in early), purple toes
- **Causes of high INR on warfarin** (1) Change in diet (2) Liver disease (3) ODEVICES (omeprazole, disulfiram, erythromycin, valproate, isoniazid, ciprofloxacin/cimetidine, acute ethanol, sulphonamide) (4) cranberry juice, (5) NSAIDs (inhibit platelet function and displace warfarin from plasma albumin) **Note PCBRAS decrease effectiveness of warfarin (phenytoin, carbamazepine, barbituates, rifampicin, chronic alcohol, sulphonylureas). Broccoli/spinach/kale/sprouts high in vitamin K, avoid!
- **Undergoing emergency surgery on warfarin**
  - Surgery can wait 6-8h – give 5mg vitamin K IV
  - Surgery can't wait – 25-50U/kg 4 factor prothrombin complex
  - Elective surgery – stop warfarin for 5 days
- **In a bleed – stop warfarin, restart when INR <5**
  - Major bleed– give 30U/kg PCC STAT + vitamin K 5mg IV (starts working > 6h)
  - Non-major bleed – give vitamin k 1-3mg IV, restart when <5

- o INR >8 & no bleed – vitamin K 1-5mg PO. Repeat INR.
- o INR 5-8 & minor bleed – stop warfarin and IV vitamin K. Repeat INR.
- o INR 5-8 & no bleed – withhold 1 or 2 doses of warfarin. Repeat INR.

- When to use warfarin vs DOAC
  - o Use warfarin **CrCl<30ml/min, extracranial bleeding** (extracranial bleed), **poor compliance, weight >120kg, an arterial thrombosis**
  - O Use DOAC **non-valvular AF** (not valves), **VTE**, previous **ICH**, use of **other drugs** (frequent/intermittent/variable), **good control** (TTR >65%).

7. RHEUMATOLOGY

GENERAL TIPS

- One should differentiate the different types of presentation of arthritis based on clinical stem.

- Autoantibody matching in the EMQs are a favourite.

- You should be able to recognise and manage rheumatological emergencies e.g., septic arthritis, GCA, and scleroderma renal crisis

ARTHRITIS

- *Osteoarthritis* – Old, Obese, trauma. Oligo/pauci-arthritis (< 5 joints) and can be asymmetrical. At **DIPJ (HerbeDen nodes) and PIPJ (Bouchard nodes).** Joint stiffness worsen throughout day (with use) + crepitus + muscle wasting +/- neuropathic pain from osteophytes. **Tx:** ladder -> lifestyle/conservative w paracetamol -> NSAID -> co-codamol -> intra-articular steroids injection -> joint replacement

- *Rheumatoid arthritis* – universal + smoking + FHx. Poly-arthritis (> 5 joints), symmetrical and **deforming**. Inflammation – constitutional Sx with joint early morning stiffness and pain **improving with use** (gelling phenomenon). Joints are boggy + rheumatoid nodules (S/C lumps; associated with 100% RhF seropositivity)
  - Patterns: 70% insidious, 15% acute (waves of stiffness and pain in young women), 10% systemic (constitutional), 5% palindromic (migrating)
  - **Systemic associations:** ILD, pleural effusion, atherosclerosis, anaemia, mononeuritis multiplex + compression neuropathy, scleritis (painful) + episcleritis (superficial redness), vasculitic ulcers, **Felty syndrome (RA +splenomegaly +neutropenia)**, higher risk of lymphoma
  - Deformities:
    - Swan-neck deformity → DIPJ flexed, PIPJ hyperextended
    - Boutonniere deformity → PIPJ flexed, DIPJ hyperextended
    - Z-thumb → MCPJ fixed flexion & P+DIPJ hyperextended
    - Jaccoud's arthropathy – ulnar subluxation (NON-erosive)
    - Vaughan-Jackson – cannot extend little finger due to extensor tendon disruption that begins on ulnar side.
    - Arthritis mutilans – destructive joint disease
    - Atlanto-axial deformity (C-spine at risk during intubation)

- Dx:

ACR 1987 – useful for taking history	ACR/EULAR 2010 - useful for diagnosis
Rheumatoid factor	Anti-CCP and rheumatoid factor ➤ Both negative = 0 ➤ Low positive either = +2 ➤ High positive either = +3
	Elevated ESR/CRP ➤ +1
Number of joints (hands and ≥ 3)	Joint involvement (large jt.– all else; small jt.– hands, wrists, feet) ➤ >10 small = +5 ➤ 4-10 small = +3 ➤ 1-3 small = +2 ➤ 2-10 large = +1 (1 large = 0)
	> 6 weeks criteria ➤ +1

Old criteria now removed: XR, symmetry, rheumatoid nodules, and EMS

- Rheumatoid Factor = IgM vs Fc portion of IgG (70% +ve in RA)
- XR signs: **osteopenia** (darker on XR), cartilage loss, space loss, **erosions**, subluxation
- DAS28 activity strata- # jt swollen, # tender, patient experience, ESR/CRP
- Management: DAS > 5.1 → start steroids AND conventional DMARDs (MTX+HCQ), review in 6-9 months (aim < 2.6).
  - If DAS > 5.1 **and** already on2. DMARDs, add biologic DMARDs.

- Psoriatic arthritis (HLA-B27)
  - Can present as ANY joint pattern.
  - Psoriatic rash (itchy, symmetrical, well-defined silvery scaly plaques on elbows, knees, scalp: extensors surfaces; Koebnernisation)
  - Tendon disease → Achilles tenditis, golfer and tennis elbows, plantar fasciitis, and dactylitis (sausage finger due to synovitis and tendon involvement)
  - Nail disease (pitting, onycholysis, subungual hyperkeratosis, dystrophy) predict joint problem.
  - Tests: ESR, XR (terminal phalanx mottling; pencil-in-cup deformity; NO erosions or osteopenia c.f. RA). **Seronegative spondyloarthropathy**
  - Tx – **NSAIDs & MTX (avoid steroids:** psoriatic flare); SSZ in spinal or peripheral disease; *severe cases* – ciclopsorin, retinoids, anti-TNF, anti-IL-17 (secukinumab), joint IL-12 and IL-23 blocker (ustenkinumab)
- Reactive arthritis (HLA-B27)
  - Reiter's syndrome: Can't see (uveitis), can't pee (urethritis/cervicitis), can't climb a tree (joint pain – usually **MONOarthopathy**)
  - Special mucocutaneous rashes: **keratoderma blenorrhagia** – palmoplantar pustular rash; **circinate balanitis** – rash around urethral meatus, behind foreskin
  - Commonly associated bugs: *Salmonella, Chlamydia, Campylobacter.* **NOT gonococcal – causes septic arthritis instead. Seronegative spondyloarthropathy.**

- o   Tx: self-limiting (NSAIDs +/- steroid injection, no Abx)
- Ankylosing spondylitis (HLA-B27)
    - o   Sacro-iliac joints and spine inflammation (LBP) in young adult males
    - o   Disease of "A"s
        - ▪   Achilles tenditis, anterior uveitis, aortitis (AR), apical pulmonary fibrosis, acute pleural effusion, anterior chest wall fusion, and associated colitis
    - o   Tests: **radiological evidence needed** (XR spine: early sacroiliitis → Romano lesion → syndesmophytes → end-stage bamboo spine); **seronegative spondyloarthropathy**
    - o   1st line Tx: **stop smoking**, NSAIDs + early PT
    - o   2nd line: Anti-TNFα
    - o   3rd line: secukinumab

- Crystal arthropathies

Gout	Red meat, EtOH, thiazides and thiazide-like (indapamide) precipitate attacks.
	Dx → Joint aspiration: **negatively birefringent needle-shaped MSU crystals.**
	Tx → NSAID 1st line → colchicine (NSAID untolerated or on A/C) → steroids
	F/U in 4-6 weeks to check BP; serum uric acid; HbA1C, renal, lipid profile.
	PPx → Urate Lowering Therapy (ULT): allopurinol (shouldn't be started acutely as prolongs, but should NOT be stopped; start once acute attack resolve).
	Start low (50-100) and titrate every 4 weeks until serum uric acid < 300 1st 3m. eGFR-dependent dosage: low-dose 50 mg OD.
	S/E: rashes common (rarely SJS), somnolence, vertigo, ataxia.
	2nd line = Febuxostat (LFT before starting). Titrate 4 weeks.
	Consider Rx colchicine > low-dose NSAID before initiating or increase dose as risk of ppt acute attack. ULTs are lifelong...
Pseudogout	M>W before age 50.
	Calcium pyrophosphate dihydrate (CPPD) ➔ rhomboid +ve birefringement
	XR – **chondrocalcinosis** (CPPD crystals)
	Large jt = shoulder, wrist, knee.
	Attacks more prolonged than gout but less painful.
	Tx = NSAIDs (colchicine if C/I), rest, local injection.

- Septic arthritis – red hot MONOarthropathy + patient unwell. Aspirate + IV Abx. May need washout.

DMARDs

- **Methotrexate** – <u>teratogenic</u> + requires folate replacement (it is a folate antagonist). S/E: pneumonitis/ILD, GI upset, bone marrow suppression, hepatotoxicity. Monitor FBC, LFT, CXR, Cr at baseline.
- **Sulphasalazine** – bone marrow suppression (FBC monitoring), hepatotoxic (LFTs), rash, and *male infertility*.
- **Hydroxychloroquine** – BULLSEYE'S maculopathy (yearly screen if > 40 y or previous ocular problem)
- **Azathioprine** – fever, bruising, hepatotoxicity, bone marrow suppression (LFTs, FBC at baseline)
- **Penicillamine** – drug-induced SLE, rash, ulcers, taste loss, proteinuria (check protein:Cr ratio), bone marrow suppression (FBC)
- **Cyclophosphamide** – skin pigmentation, *male infertility*, **haemorrhagic cystitis**
- **Ciclosporin** – bone marrow suppression, <u>renal failure</u> (hyperK+, Cr, hypertension, oedema), gingival hyperplasia
- **Anti-TNFa**
    - Screen for TB beforehand → can cause disseminated TB from reactivation
    - Other S/E: CHF, sepsis, demyelination

CONNECTIVE TISSUE DISEASES

<u>SLE</u>

- Dx 4/17 SLICC criteria (1 clinical + 1 immunological)

- Clinical
  1. Acute cutaneous – "malar"
  2. Chronic cutaneous – discoid etc.
  3. Non-scarring alopecia
  4. Oronasal ulcers
  5. Arthritis ($\geq$ 2 joints) – wrists, knees, PIPJ
  6. Serositis – pleuritis, pericarditis
  7. Renal – **most common type IV nephritis** (diffuse proliferative GN), others (e.g. type V = membranous → only one that is nephrotic).
  8. Neuropsychiatric
  9. Haemolytic anaemia (severe disease; **type II HS**)
  10. Leukopenia
  11. Thrombocytopenia (< 100; severe disease)

- Immunological
  1. DCT +ve (don't count again if AIHA)
  2. ANA
  3. Anti-DNA
  4. Anti-Smith (RNP) – <u>not</u> SM
  5. Antiphospholipid antibodies
  6. Low C' (C3, C4, CH50)

- **Antibodies:**
  - ANA is dilutional (the higher the denominator, the more positive it is; cut-off 1:80)
  - Double-stranded DNA – high specificity, correlate with activity.
  - Anti-Smith – 100% specificity, very insensitive. Severe and renal disease.
  - Ro/La, U1-RNP, anti-phospholipid
  - Drug-induced lupus (penicillamine, isoniazid, minocycline, hydralazine, phenytoin, procainamide, quinidine, and anti-TNFα) → **anti-histone; reversible when drug stop**

APS: 1/3 of SLE cases (mainly primary)
Mixture of anti-cardiolipin, anti-beta2 glycoprotein1, and "lupus anticoagulant"
Hypercoagulable state = recurrent pregnancy loss, DVTs, PEs, MI, Budd-Chiari syndrome, strokes.
Lab = *paradoxically long APTT due to interference by* Lupus anticoagulant
Dx criteria = **APS Ab on 2 separate occasions 12 weeks apart <u>AND</u>** thrombosis *OR* pregnancy morbidity (once > 10/40, once premie < 34/40, or 3X < 10/40)
Tx = HCQ, AZA, low-dose steroids (safe in pregnancy) **and** anticoagulation (LMWH during pregnancy, warfarin lifelong)

- SLE Tx:
  - General – avoid sunlight
  - Mild – NSAID + hydroxychloroquine (reduces flare, increase survival, anti-thrombotic)
  - Moderate – hydroxychloroquine + low-dose steroids $\pm$ AZA/MTX (if difficulty tapering steroids)

- o Severe – pulse steroids, MMF, cyclophosphamide, biologics
- o In SLE who are pregnant, aspirin 75 mg should be given to reduce pre-eclampsia risk

Sjögren's
- Female, middle-aged, autoimmune begets autoimmune
- 2 out of 3: presentation (sicca, xerostomia, dry vagina = thrush + dyspareunia); labs (anti-RNP = anti-Ro (SSA)/ anti-La (SSB) in 60%), or biopsy of <u>small</u> salivary glands (CD4 T-cell infiltration; avoid parotid gland – risk CN VII damage)
- Other tests: RhF (100%), ANA, high ESR, Schirmer's test (<5 mm in 5 mins), sialometry
- **Complications:** (1) higher risk of B-cell marginal zone lymphoma, (2) neonatal lupus
- **Tx:** symptomatic, NSAID, HCQ...

Neonatal lupus
Anti-Ro > anti-La can cross the placenta and lead to congenital heart block

Polymyositis and dermatomyositis

- POLYmyositis → skeletal muscle only
- DERMATOmyositis → skin + skeletal muscle involvement.

MUSCLE
- **B/L proximal muscle weakness**
- **TENDER to palpation**
- **Esp. anti-gravity muscles**
- **"Can't comb hair, can't climb stairs, can't hang laundry, can't reach upper shelves, stuck in bathtub"**
- **Waddling gait (can't stabilise bilaterally during swing phase of gait)**

SKIN
- **Shawl sign**
- **Heliotrope rash**
- **Gottron's papule**
- **Linear erythema**
- **Angioedema**
- **Mechanic's hand**
- **Hyperaemic nail fold, capillary loop dilatation**

- ANA+, anti-Jo1 (20% in myositis, associated with ILD), high CK
- Other tests: EMG, T2 MRI (oedema = hyperintensity), biopsy
- Tx: steroids, IVIg, rituximab, cyclophosphamide
- **Red flags:** muscle burnout (a falling CK may mean all muscle has been lost rather than recovery), SOB (multifactorial – weak muscles of chest wall, ILD, bulbar weakness leading to aspiration pneumonia), *suspect cancer* (screen in > 40y with dermatomyositis and up to 5-years post-Dx).

Systemic sclerosis

- Limited subtype = CREST (Calcinosis/**anti-Centromere**, Raynaud's, Esophageal dysmotility, Sclerodactyly, Telangiectasia of face) → face, elbow, knees, feet (sparing trunk). **More associated with pulmonary hypertension**.
- Diffuse subtype = skin tightening affecting neck and trunk with **early organ involvement (ILD > pulm hypertension)**, cardiac fibrosis, GI dysmotility, renal crisis (hypertension Tx by **ACE inhibitors**). **Anti-Scl70 (topoisomerase I).**
- **Tx:** cyclophosphamide for severe disease

VASCULITIS

<u>Small vessel vasculitis</u>
- ANCA – anti-nuclear cytoplasmic antibody; detected by immunofluorescence in 2 patterns: c-ANCA and p-ANCA; or via ELISA.

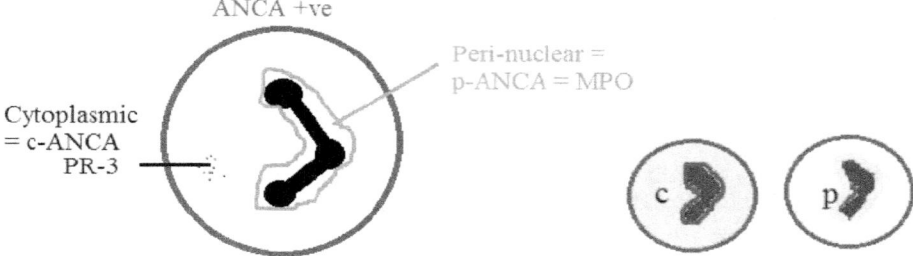

- Differentials of pulmonary renal-syndromes = **haemoptysis and haematuria PLUS:**
  - Wegener's (GPA) – cavitating lung lesions + ENT/nasopharyngeal Sx. Relapsing necrotising <u>G</u>ranulomatous vasculitic disease of "C"s
    - Chest/lungs = haemoptysis + Cavitating lesions of lung or bilateral ifniltrates
    - Crescenteric rapid progressive glomerulonephritis
    - C-ANCA/CRP
    - Cyclophosphamide/Corticosteroids
    - Can't walk = arthalgia
    - Can't hear = deafness (otitis media, CN VIII, mononeuritis
    - Can't breathe = tracheal stenosis (requires tracheostomy), nasal septum destruction (like Cocaine)
  - MPA → palpable purpura = vasculitic rash. Tx similar to GPA. Non-granulomatous, relapse vasculitis of "**P**"s:
    - **P**ulmonary haemorrhage
    - **P**roteinruia
    - **P**alpable purpura + vasculitis rash
    - **P**eripheral neuropathy
    - **P**olyarthalgia
    - **P**ainful gut (mesenteric angina)
    - **P**-ANCA
  - Lupus → 4/17 of SLICC criteria
  - Goodpasture → type IV collagen antibodies against glomerular basement membrane (anti-GBM) → rapid-onset ("crescenteric") nephritis, *simultaneous* with lung collagen (type IV) damage. **Dx:** anti-GBM, +/-ANCA, Bx. **Tx:** plasma exchange, cyclophosphamide (can also cause hamaturia), rituximab (reduce autoantibody production), and transplant.
  - Others e.g., IgA nephropathy and HSP (post URTI)
- **Churg-Strauss = eosinophilic granulomatosis with polyangiitis**
  - **Small-medium** vessel vasculitis
  - Adult-onset asthma (DDx: carcinoid) w nasal polyps (2/3 Samter's triad)
  - Eosinophilia (DDx: atopy, helminths), IgE

- o Eosiniphilic pneumonia + heart involvement
  - o ANCA may be positive but unrelated to disease activity
- Cryoglobulinaemia
  - o Insoluble proteins, usually Ig, that precipitate at low temperatures
  - o Type 1 = monoclonal (IgG/M) or their light chains → therefore, seen in MGUS-myeloma spectrum, CLL/Waldenström hyperglobulinaemia
    - Pt: hyperviscosity syndrome = headache, visual/hearing changes, palpable purpura, acrocyanosis, Raynaud's, *livedo reticularis = net-like lacy purple rash on the legs in the cold*, signs of high output heart failure
  - o Type 2 = hep C associated
  - o Type 3 = "mixed" polyclonal IgG/M/A disease → associated with autoimmune (begets autoimmune) and hep C
  - o **Cryoglobulin tests must be sent in special flask at 37°C, or drawn**
    - Other tests: RhF (much higher than RA as Ig precipitated out).
  - o Tx: steroids + cyclophosphamide → plasma exchange

NOT to be confused by cold agglutinins:
Autoimmune haemolytic anaemia that occurs in the cold due to cold-activated autoAb to RBC antigens. Pt: peripheral cyanosis + liveo reticularis + anaemia (= pallor/jaundiced, tired, SOB) that improves in the warm
Associated: Mycoplasma, EBV, CMV, HIV

Medium vessel vasculitis
- Polyarteritis nodosa - all organs affected by necrotitising vasculitis **except** lungs
  - Coronary -> angina
  - Renal -> AKI + HTN
  - SMA -> mesenteric angina = post-prandial colicky pain
  - Skin ulcers, livedo reticularis
  - Neuro – mononeuritis multiplex (vasa nervosum inflammation)
  - Myalgia
  - Sterile orchitis in male (recurrent testicular pain, not resolved by Abx)
  - Dx: Bx and angiogram (saccular micronauerysms w alternating fibrosis)
  - **Associated with Hep B surface Ag**
  - Tx: mild → AZA, MTX, MMF → cyclophosphamide → once inflammation settle, can stent areas of fibrosis (do not stent whilst inflamed as can rupture)

Large vessel vasculitis
- **Takayasu arteritis**
  - Claudication in patients who do not deserve to (young, Asian, females, non-vasculopath).
  - O/E: pulseless disease, subclavian bruit
  - Dx: radiological (MRA or CT-PET)
  - Tx: pulse steroids + cyclophosphamide – stent once inflammation dampened

- Giant cell /temporal arteritis
  - Granulomatous inflammation – predilection of extracranial branches of carotid artery → constitutional Sx; pulse-synchronous pulsing headache (unilateral)
  - Stiff, tender temporal artery; scalp tenderness w facial pain
  - **Jaw claudication** (masseter fatigue), arm claudication
  - Vertigo and hearing loss
  - Amaurosis fugax/painless transient visual loss (due to arteritic anterior ischaemic optic neuropathy of the posterior ciliary artery)
  - Polymyalgia rheumatica (= muscle-ache w early morning stiffness of shoulder and hip girdles).
  - Dx: clinical... low pickup of skip lesions do not rule out Dx
  - Tx: pulse steroids (IV then PO) first-line (without waiting for Bx)

Printed in Great Britain
by Amazon

21004203R00058